D0783086

What is acupressure?

Thousands of years ago, the Chinese made a chance discovery that was to lead to a method of healing which is just as effective in the 1980's as it was in 300 B.C. The discovery was that pain and illness could be relieved by puncturing or pressing certain points on the body. They made up a 'map' of all these points, and so acupuncture and acupressure came into being.

Acupressure is acupuncture without needles. It is safe, painless and, unlike some of the drugs on the market today, it has no side-effects. Pain, illness and psychological problems can be successfully treated by acupressure. It can be used alone or in conjunction with other methods of treatment. And the beauty of it is that you can treat yourself at home. Once your doctor has diagnosed your complaint and you have discussed your course of treatment with him, you can use this book to carry out your acupressure programme.

Dr Frank Bahr, one of Europe's leading medically qualified acupressure experts, describes the pressure points for a variety of ailments, and explains the methods of treatment for each. Location of the points is helped by 300 illustrations which show the points and the direction in which to massage them. And the book includes treatment by ear-acupressure, a new dimension which has been developed during the last twenty years.

With its section on emergency treatments, its alphabetical arrangement of ailments and its clear style and comprehensive illustrations, this book is a practical layman's guide to health.

By the Same Author
The Acupressure Slimming Book

THE ACUPRESSURE HEALTH BOOK

Frank Bahr

Translated from the German by
Philip Dale
in association with
First Edition

London
UNWIN PAPERBACKS
Boston   Sydney

First published in Great Britain in Unwin Paperbacks 1982

This book is copyright under the Berne Convention.
No reproduction without permission. All rights reserved.

UNWIN® PAPERBACKS
40 Museum Street, London, WC1A 1LU, UK

Unwin Paperbacks,
P.O. Box 18, Park Lane, Hemel Hempstead, Herts HP2 4TE, UK

George Allen & Unwin Australia Pty Ltd.,
8 Napier Street, North Sydney, NSW 2060, Australia

German Edition *Akupressur: Erfolgreiche Selbstbehandlung
bei Schmerzen und Beschwerden*

© Mosaik Verlag GmbH, Munich, 1976
English translation © George Allen & Unwin (Publishers) Ltd 1982

British Library Cataloguing in Publication Data

Bahr, Frank
      The acupressure health book.
1. Acupressure
2. Self-care, Health
I. Title   II. Akupressur, Erfolgreiche
Selbstbehandlung bei Schmerzen und Beschwerden.
English
615.8'22   RM723.A27
ISBN 0-04-613044-6

Photographs: Frank Müller-May

Set in 11 on 12 point Souvenir by Fotographics (Bedford) Ltd,
and printed in Hong Kong by Dah Hua Printing Press Co., Ltd.

*To Dr P. F. M. Nogier
in recognition of his pioneering discoveries
and the importance of his scientific research.*

Contents

ABC of pains and illnesses   *page*   7

Introduction   11

What is acupressure?   11

What is acupressure for?   11

The relief of pain   11

Functional disorders and psychological problems   12

The cure without side effects   12

Acupressure as a protective measure   12

Acupressure for improved physical performance   13

Emergency treatment   14

How acupressure evolved   14

How to find the right acupressure points   15

Choosing the right acupressure movement   15

Method and duration   16

How to use your fingers for acupressure   17

A warning against self-diagnosis   17

Suitable and unsuitable cases for treatment   17

The science of acupressure   18

Acupressure applications   22

Addresses   160

ABC of pains and illnesses

(Chapter headings are in colour)

Addictions   22
Amputations – *see* Phantom limb   122
Angina pectoris – *see* Emergency
   acupressure   62
Anxiety   24
Appendicitis – *see* Emergency acupressure   58
Appetite   26
Arms, circulation – *see* Circulation
   disorders   38
Arm and shoulder pains   28
Arthritis – *see* Knee pains   96
Arthrosis – *see* Knee pains   96
Asthma attacks – *see* Emergency
   acupressure   56

Bedwetting   30
Belching   32
Bladder disorders   34
Blue lips – *see* Heart weakness   82
Bowel action – *see* Diarrhoea – and
   Constipation   46, 54
Brain, circulation – *see* Circulation
   disorders   40
Bronchitis – *see* Coughs and bronchitis   50

Catarrh – *see* Colds and catarrh   44
Cerebellum – *see* Vertigo   156
Cervical vertebrae, disorders of the – *see* Spinal
   complaints   138
Circulation disorders of the arms and
   hands   38
Circulation disorders of the brain   40
Circulation disorders of the feet and legs   42
Coccyx, disorders of the – *see* Spinal
   complaints   138
Colds and catarrh   44
Colic – *see* Emergency acupressure   56
Concentration, lack of – *see* Forgetfulness   70
Constipation   46
Coronary thrombosis – *see* Emergency
   acupressure   62

Coughs and bronchitis   50
Cystitis – *see* Bladder disorders   34

Depression   52
Despair – *see* Depression   52
Diarrhoea   54
Digestive juices – *see* Pancreatic problems   120
Disturbed sleep – *see* Sleeping problems   134

Early morning sickness – *see* Nausea   112
Emergency acupressure   56
Energy, lack of – *see* Keeping fit   92
Examination stress – *see* Anxiety   24

Feet, circulation – *see* Circulation
   disorders   42
Flatulence   68
Forgetfulness and lack of concentration   70
Frigidity – *see* Sex   128

Gall bladder malfunction   72
Gall bladder colic – *see* Emergency
   acupressure   60
Gastric ulcers – *see* Stomach pains   146
Giddiness – *see* Vertigo   156

Haemorrhoids (Piles)   74
Hands, circulation – *see* Circulation
   disorders   38
Hay fever   76
Headaches – *see* Migraine   100
Hearing defects   78
Heartbeat, irregular – *see* Heart
   palpitations   80
Heart pains – *see* Emergency acupressure   62
Heart palpitations   80
Heart weakness   82
Hip pains   84

Hoarseness   86
Hormonal imbalance – see Migraine   100
Hormonal troubles in women   88
Hot flushes – see Hormonal troubles   88

Impotence – see Sex   128
Intestinal cramp – see constipation   46
Intestinal gas – see Flatulence   68
Irritability – see Nervousness   114

Keeping fit   92
Kidney malfunction   94
Kidney pains – see Emergency
    acupressure   56
Knee pains   96

Labyrinth of the ear – see Vertigo   156
Legs, circulation – see Circulation
    disorders   42
Liver trouble   98
Loneliness – see Depression   52
Lumbar vertebrae, disorders of the – see Spinal
    complaints   138

Memory weakness – see Forgetfulness   70
Menopausal problems – see Hormonal
    troubles   88
Menstrual irregularities – see Hormonal
    troubles   88
Migraine   100
Mouth, inflammation of the lining   110

Nausea, travel sickness and early morning
    sickness   112
Nervousness and irritability   114
Nettle rash – see Skin allergies   130

Nightmares – see Sleeping problems   134
Nose bleeds   116
Nystagmus – see Vertigo   156

Otogenous vertigo – see Vertigo   156
Overfull feeling   118
Overwork – see Keeping fit   92

Pancreatic problems   120
Peptic ulcers – see Stomach pains   146
Phantom limb   122
Piles – see Haemorrhoids   74
Prostate gland, inflammation of the   124

Sacrum, disorders of the – see Spinal
    complaints   138
Sciatica   126
Sex – stimulating sexual activity   128
Shoulder pains – see Arm and shoulder
    pains   28
Sickness, early morning – see Nausea   112
Sickness, travel – see Nausea   112
Skin allergies and nettle rash   130
Skin irritation   132
Sleeping problems   134
Smoker's cough – see Coughs and
    bronchitis   50
Sneezing – see Hay fever   76
Speech disorders – see Stuttering   148
Spinal complaints   138
Stomach pains and gastric or peptic
    ulcers   146
Stress – see Keeping fit   92
Stuttering   148
Swallowing air – see Belching 32 and
    Flatulence 68

Tennis elbow   150
Thoracic vertebrae, disorders of the – see Spinal
    complaints   138
Tonsillitis   152
Toothache – see Emergency acupressure   66
Tranquillizers – see Anxiety   24
Travel sickness – see Nausea   112

Ulcers – see Stomach pains   146

Varicose veins   154
Vertigo (Giddiness)   156

Introduction

What is acupressure?

The stimulation of acupressure points is the oldest and most widespread healing method in the world. The Chinese are credited with discovering, thousands of years ago, that internal complaints could be cured or relieved through points on the outside of the body, and today there are various methods of treating these points. The oldest and simplest of these is concentrated massage, otherwise known as acupressure. The application of needles is known as acupuncture, and there are other forms of stimulation, involving the use of heat, ultrasonic waves, laser beams, underwater massage jets, and so on.

What is acupressure for?

Acupressure and acupuncture are now taught at a number of universities throughout the world and, as a result of the successes achieved, more and more doctors are taking training courses in classical acupuncture (of the body); the newer form, ear acupuncture (auricular medicine – from the Latin *auricula*, meaning ear); and acupressure. Whereas acupuncture should only be carried out by a properly trained doctor, the patient himself can use the acupressure method, which is easy to learn and to apply. For these reasons, and because of the growing sense of responsibility of the individual for his own health and well-being, acupressure is arousing widespread interest among the general public, especially since it has none of the side effects which drugs often produce, and it costs nothing. Any health-conscious reader will immediately recognize the value of acupressure in such cases as:

the relief of complaints relating to body functions and persistent ailments,

pain relief until the arrival of a doctor or admission into hospital,

protection against a relapse following an earlier illness,

supplementing a course of treatment prescribed and supervised by a doctor,

improving physical performance,

first aid in cases of emergency.

The relief of pain

The *History of Chinese Acupuncture and Moxibustion* (the application of heat to acupuncture points), which was published in China in 1975, states 'Acupressure to points of the ear or other parts of the body relieves pain.' During my own visits to China to study acupuncture, in 1974, 1975 and 1976, I was able to satisfy myself that this process is not just confined to books, but is widely practised in universities, and by people at home, including children.

Pain is the body's warning signal, so acupressure should only be applied after accurate diagnosis. Admittedly, knowing what causes the pain – whether it be in the form of repeated headaches, chronic back pains due to worn spinal discs, persistent knee pains due to arthritic joints, or whatever – does not make it any easier to bear. But a different aspect of pain is mentioned by Dr Nogier in his textbook on auricular therapy (ear acupuncture), when he says, 'We should avoid eliminating pain altogether if it is necessary for the purpose of following the course of an illness or indicating the need for an operation.' Practice acupressure in consultation with your doctor, and save on drugs and medicine.

11

Functional disorders and psychological problems

Following its successful use for the treatment of pain, accupressure began to be used, thousands of years ago, for other things, such as circulation problems and stimulating the proper functioning of the organs. Subsequently, it has come to be used in the treatment of psychological illnesses and its fields of application have consequently grown considerably, as may be seen from the contents of this book alone. The same advice applies in these circumstances as it does in the treatment of pain: use acupressure only after accurate diagnosis. If you do so in consultation with your doctor you will soon be able to reduce your intake of drugs.

The cure without side effects

There is much talk nowadays about the harmful, and even dangerous, effects of drugs which were once considered perfectly safe. Thalidomide used to be thought a harmless sleeping pill, and Phenacetin a safe cure for headaches, but today it is recognized that the former, when taken during pregnancy, was responsible for a number of cases of deformity in babies, while the latter could cause severe kidney trouble. In current medical journals it is strongly argued that the sale of drugs, originally considered harmless, should be stopped, as in the recent case of a laxative widely sold in Japan, whose manufacturer paid out $250 million in compensation to those affected. There is a similar case over a slimming drug in America. The long list of drugs withdrawn from sale is being steadily extended without receiving very much public attention. Even doctors themselves make very little of such matters, so as not to give their patients cause for alarm. However, it would be unwise to turn against all drugs,

without differentiating between them. This is true even of medicines with pronounced side effects, if the doctor prescribes them after careful consideration of all the aspects of the case. In many instances, a patient using acupressure needs less drugs, and can often do without them altogether after a time.

Any reduction should only be made in consultation with the doctor treating the case, but it is obviously beneficial if the patient can cut down on his drug intake through the use of acupressure. Of course, for certain illnesses, the drug intake should not be reduced and acupressure only serves to improve the patient's condition; if he has a weak heart for instance.

Acupressure as a protective measure

Acupressure not only relieves pain and illness, it also protects against illness, which makes it of great benefit to health generally. Nowadays, about 80 per cent of medical practice is of a so-called 'curative' nature; that is, the treatment of existing illnesses. Among those who look to the future, however, it is generally agreed that, within the next ten years, preventative treatment, which provides protection against the onset of illness, will increase from its present level of 20 per cent to 80 per cent, and curative medicine will be needed in only the remaining 20 per cent of cases. This is desirable, not only from the point of view of health, but also from that of nations' economies, because enormous sums of money can be saved by this method. Evidence of this is already to be seen in protective measures against cancer, and in influenza injections. This has long been the case in China where, to quote from the textbook previously mentioned, 'Clinical experience has shown that acupressure or acupuncture, applied to appropriate points, offers protection against certain illnesses.' The West will also find acupressure taking its place as an effective and inexpensive protective measure. Visiting politicians to China will undoubtedly bring back some of the 'Chinese wisdom' with them, and lend support to the use of acupressure on political grounds.

Acupressure for improved physical performance

(the method used by world and Olympic champions)

'Nothing has helped me so much recently as acupressure.' Statements of this kind by the high jumper Dwight Stones, and the discus thrower Mac Wilkins, both world record holders at their respective events, caused a sensation at the Montreal Olympics of 1976. But this method of improving an athlete's performance – a method which is both safe and beneficial – is not a new one. It is in fact so old that it is reflected in the nickname given to one of the Chinese acupuncture points. This point *tsu-san-li*, in addition to its description 'great healer of feet and knees', is also known in China as 'three villages', because it increases normal walking capacity by several miles – the distances between three villages. This point is not only used by servicemen and sportsmen, but is also known to improve the performance of racehorses.

Near this point there is another, the master point of the muscular system, known in China as *yang-ling-ch'üan*. This acts against cramp, swelling, and inflammation of the muscles and tendons, and so is much used by competitive athletes.

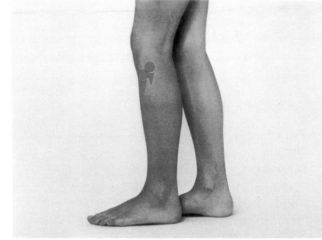

The point *tsu-san-li* has to be massaged in a downward direction. If you place your hand on top of your kneecap, you will find this point immediately below the tip of your ring finger. The point next to it is the *yang-ling-ch'uan*, which is situated just below the top of the outer legbone (fibula).

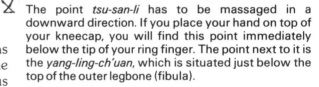

The point *nei-kuan* is situated two or three fingerwidths below the base of the palm, in the middle of the inside lower arm.

13

The heart of an athlete is put to considerable strain. This is relieved by the acupressure point called in Chinese *nei-kuan*, meaning 'internal barrier', which helps to regulate circulation and breathing, and acts against the tendency towards tension in this area. How does the specialist react to all this?

Dr Zier is a sports physician at Damp 2000, a well-known hospital and recreation centre in Germany. He is carrying out trials with acupuncture, and says, 'I have measured the performance of athletes on a cycling machine before and after the stimulation of acupuncture points. So far, in every case, there has been an increase in performance, shown by a reduction in the heartbeat of ten to thirty beats a minute, for the same amount of effort. Acupuncture also has a very good effect on muscular pain and cramp.'

It would be wrong to assume that acupressure of the points mentioned above is suitable only for athletes: it is equally suitable for all sportsmen, whatever their pursuit.

Emergency treatments

Emergencies can happen when it is not possible to reach a doctor quickly, if at all – on holiday in some inaccessible place, for example, or maybe abroad, or at sea. If there is a delay before proper medical treatment can be given, acupressure can be used as a means of first aid.

A later chapter of this book deals with emergency acupressure in cases of:

asthma attacks
acute appendicitis
gall bladder trouble
pains around the heart
kidney pains
toothache

How acupressure evolved

Several centuries before they developed the present method of stimulating acupuncture points, the Chinese made the chance discovery that pain or illness was relieved if certain places on the body were pressed or punctured. They began to treat illnesses which responded to the therapy of massaging or tapping certain localized points on the body, and gradually the pattern of acupuncture points evolved. The tapping and massaging were done with certain stones, called *zehn-shi* in Chinese, which means 'stone needle', and from these acupuncture needles were later developed.

The first written record of acupressure appears in a medical book which was compiled in the Tsin dynasty in about 300 B.C. This deals with emergency acupressure for circulation failure and the state of coma. As a result, acupressure found its way into Chinese homes as a form of first aid. (From the *History of Chinese Acupuncture and Moxibustion*, published in China in 1975.)

Ear acupressure, on the other hand, was not developed in China, but in Lyons, by Dr Paul Nogier. At that time only a few points of the ear were known and the exact relationship between them and the individual parts of the body and organs had not been discovered, until, in 1957, Dr Nogier's publications drew public attention to the method. Subsequently, he and his team evolved a complete 'map' of the ear, on which all the appropriate areas of the body were recorded. Dr Nogier not only discovered the points of the ear but also ways in which they could be stimulated.

It might be thought that the Chinese would not accept this development, as it was not their own, but the reverse was the case. In their latest book on needle analgesia, published in Shanghai in 1973, roughly half the subject matter is devoted to ear acupuncture.

How to find the right acupressure points

When practising acupressure, it is essential to find the true points. The more accurately you massage the right point, the greater the effect. The illustrations in this book show where the points are. For best results you should always use all three of the following ways to find the appropriate point:

1 Visual

Look carefully at the illustrations on the subject in question and find the point, or points, on your own body. For the points of the ear you will either need to use a mirror or get someone else to hold the illustration as close as possible to your own ear, and then transfer the point in your mind's eye.

2 Visual and manual

Read closely the sections headed 'Body acupressure' and 'Ear acupressure', in which the exact location of each point is described. Place the appropriate number of fingers across the body, starting at the reference point, and then locate the corresponding acupressure point.

3 Sensitivity

As a final check, you need to know that each point is more sensitive to pressure than the surrounding area. This means that pressure from the fingers is felt more strongly there than on the flesh around it.

Sometimes you will need help to find the points on the back. In order to locate these accurately, you should count the vertebrae. This may sound difficult but the seventh cervical vertebra – the lowest in the neck – is usually easy to see and feel due to its prominent appearance (hence its Latin name, *vertebra prominens*). The helper should mark this point with a felt-tipped pen. The patient then bends over, throwing the spinal column into greater relief, so that each vertebra can be counted. The first twelve are the thoracic vertebrae, below which are five lumbar vertebrae. If difficulties occur in finding the points of the back corresponding to the treatment, a doctor should be asked to point out the exact position. Once this has been done, the patient can find the point again by making appropriate measurements –for example, 23cm below the hairline, or 15cm below the seventh vertebra and two to three finger-widths to one side. In practice, this is much easier than it sounds, because the points are noticeably sensitive to pressure, and the patient will feel whether the right point is being massaged or not.

Choosing the right acupressure movement

In China, the direction of massage is clearly laid down for all acupressure points, since each one lies on a 'one way' energy line, or 'meridian'. According to the Chinese, acupressure applied in the wrong direction has no effect whatsoever. In a widely published book issued by the University Clinic of the Medical College of Tsingtao, the direction of massage is indicated in drawings with an arrow (Fig. 1). In *The Acupressure Health Book*, the correct direction is given in both the text and the illustrations. Where several points lie close together, the arrow at the head of the row applies to all of them, and they may be massaged in one comprehensive movement.

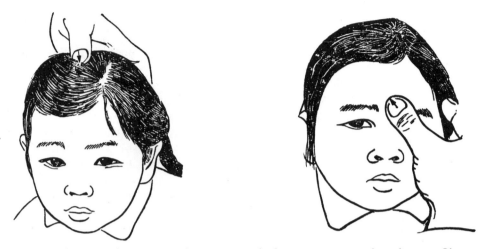

Fig. 1. *Illustration showing the correct direction in which to massage, taken from a Chinese book on acupressure. Massage applied in the wrong direction is ineffective.*

Method and duration

The amount of pressure should be the same in each case, but it may vary according to the type of complaint and the patient's age. It can be applied for longer to increase the effect, but the Chinese recommend that the total time for each day's acupressure session should be:

newborn babies: $\frac{1}{2}$–3 minutes
babies of 3–6 months: 1–4 minutes
babies of 6–12 months: 1–5 minutes
children aged 1–3 years: 3–7 minutes
older children: 5–10 minutes
adults: 5–10–15 minutes

If in doubt, you should seek the advice of a qualified acupuncturist, especially if your own efforts at acupressure fail to achieve the desired results. It may be that natural left-handers have problems, because their brain centre lies on the opposite side from that of someone who is right-handed. In such cases, patients should omit ear acupressure, and carry out body acupressure only.

The frequency of treatment depends on the type and severity of the complaint. Under each heading you will find an indication as to the number of times per day – or, after the acute stage has passed, per week – that acupressure should be applied. In general, it is best to practice ear acupressure and body acupressure on alternate days, as stated in the text. **When applying body acupressure, you should always massage the points on** *both* **sides of the body.**

The following guidelines should also be observed:

1. The room temperature should not be too hot or too cold.
2. Make sure that the air is fresh. Do not work in a stale or smoky atmosphere.
3. Sit, or lie, in a comfortable position. Do not

work with cold hands. If necessary, warm them by rubbing them together before starting.

4. Massage should be applied with rapid movements, about 70 to 100 times a minute.
5. If the patient has sensitive skin, a little massage oil or talcum powder may be used.
6. Some patients sweat freely after treatment. In this case, an interval should be allowed between each massage. On cold or windy days, the patient should wrap up warmly afterwards before going out.

How to use your fingers for acupressure

In most cases you can use the nail of your index finger, taking care to massage the points in the given direction. The fingernail should be at a right-angle to your skin.

About 30 movements in 10 seconds are normally enough. Massage the skin with your fingernail in short strokes, approximately an inch long.

If you find it easier, in the narrow parts of the ear you can use the nail of the little finger instead, or the rounded end of a pencil or a ball point pen.

The pressure on the points of the body or ear should be strong enough to be clearly felt – remember, the point must be stimulated – but not so strong as to produce red or blue marks. The pressure should be such that the skin is reddened after 30 massage strokes, but the skin surface must not be injured.

A warning against self-diagnosis

Acupressure is a very effective and completely harmless method of curing or relieving illnesses and other ailments, the great advantage being that the patient treats himself.

It could be said that no one knows his own body better than the patient, but this is not necessarily the case. It may well be true of unpleasant but relatively harmless complaints, such as persistent headaches or severe constipation, but a prolonged period of coughing, for example, should not be seen in the same light. What the patient cannot know is that some form of lung cancer may have developed which, if diagnosed in time, might respond to appropriate treatment. The same applies to stomach pains which may be due to cancer of the stomach, and so on. The patient who attempts to diagnose his own complaint is quite likely to be wrong. It is always advisable to consult your doctor for an objective diagnosis before beginning a course of acupressure.

Suitable and unsuitable cases for treatment

A study of the contents of this book shows that acupressure can be helpful in a large number of cases, including severe conditions. It can be used as a supplementary treatment, in consultation with the doctor in charge, or as a means of preventing a relapse. There are certain illnesses however, for which it is quite unsuitable, such as any form of hereditary disease, endogenous depression, schizophrenia or cancer, or conditions requiring surgery, such as a fracture, rupture or intestinal obstruction. If in doubt, consult your doctor rather than taking a chance. This applies especially to pregnant women, on whom certain points associated with active hormones should not be massaged.

If your doctor is not very well informed about

17

acupressure and acupuncture, a list of acupuncturists can be obtained from the organizations listed on page 160.

The science of acupressure

By 1979, three million operations had taken place in China, using acupuncture as the anesthetic. According to the records, not a single death occurred as a result of this form of anesthetic. This knowledge caused something of a sensation elsewhere in the world where, for the same number of operations carried out under traditional forms of anesthetic, something like 100 deaths would be expected to occur. Meanwhile, some 5,000 operations have been performed in Germany, where the process has also been found to carry no risk for the

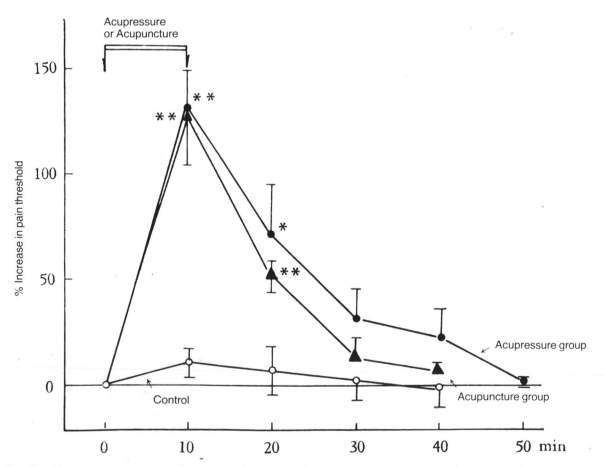

Fig. 2. *How acupuncture on the* tsu-san-li *point and acupressure on the* quen-lun *point affects the pain threshold of rabbits.*

18

patient. What is less well known is that operations that have been successfully carried out in China under acupressure include operations on the head, gynecological operations, and abdominal surgery.

For years, scientists have been working on the effectiveness of acupuncture and acupressure for the relief of pain. As a result of numerous experiments on animals, it was initially discovered that hypnosis played no part in the process. In Europe, a Dr Kothbauer successfully performed several caesarian operations on cows, using acupuncture. In America, animal clinics now exist in which both acupuncture and acupressure are used, especially in the treatment of valuable race-horses.

One of the most important establishments in China for scientific research into acupuncture and acupressure by means of animal experiments is the Peking Medical College. During my visits to China in 1974 and 1975, Dr Han Chi-sheng demonstrated on a rabbit a number of ways of reducing pain, technically known as 'raising the threshold of pain'. Fig. 2 shows how, after acupuncture of the *tsu-san-li* point, the threshold is raised by 128 per cent (line marked with triangles), and also how, after acupressure of the *quen-lun* point, at a frequency of two movements per second, it rises by a similar amount – 133 per cent (line marked with dots). As is usual with scientific experiments, a control group was tested at the same time, in order to measure variations in the threshold (line marked with circles). Each group consisted of ten rabbits. The method of applying and measuring pain during the experiment was to direct a strong ray of heat at the nostrils of a blindfolded rabbit (Fig. 3). Using a stopwatch, the researcher measured the length of time before the animal moved its head to one side, clearly indicating pain.

Later research carried out by Dr Han was even more impressive. Using sixteen rabbits, he withdrew brain fluid (*liquor cerebrospinalis*) from donor rabbits, after first raising their pain threshold by acupressure, and injected it into the brains of receiver rabbits. The latter showed a marked raising of the threshold – 82 per cent – compared with the group which had not been given acupressure (Fig. 4). This led to the conclusion that properly applied treatment brings about a change in the so-called 'neuro-transmitter' in the brain. Professor Birkmayer, Director of the Ludwig-Botsmann Institute for Neurochemistry in Vienna, has carried out research into the effect of acupuncture on the neuro-transmitter in humans, and his findings confirm those of the Chinese. Similar research is currently being done at Munich University. Dr Han also gave details about other research activities at Peking Medical College, in which electro-physiological experiments on animals showed that strong pressure on the muscles and tendons has an inhibiting effect on neural discharge in the non-specific nuclei of the

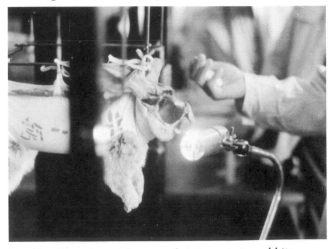

Fig. 3. *Experimental research into pain in rabbits after acupuncture or acupressure*

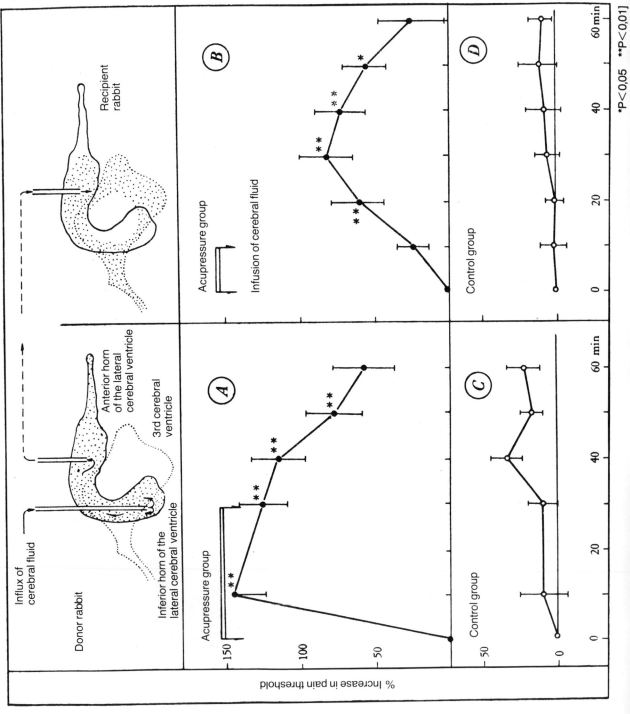

20

*P<0,05 **P<0,01

Recipient rabbit

Donor rabbit

Influx of cerebral fluid

Anterior horn of the lateral cerebral ventricle

3rd cerebral ventricle

Inferior horn of the lateral cerebral ventricle

% Increase in pain threshold

Ⓐ Acupressure group

Ⓑ Acupressure group Infusion of cerebral fluid

Ⓒ Control group

Ⓓ Control group

60 min

thalamus in rats and rabbits and the reticular formation in guineapigs.

It is impossible, in this book, to cover all the other animal experiments which have taken place under acupressure. Further information can be found in the Chinese journal, *Scientia Sinica*, English Edition, Volume 17, February 1974, which is obtainable from Guozi Shudian, China Publications Centre, P.O. Box 399, Peking, People's Republic of China.

N.B.   On the illustrations of the ear, throughout the book, 'links' means 'left', and 'rechts' means 'right'.

Fig. 4   *The effect of acupressure demonstrated by the experimental transfer of brain fluid*

ACUPRESSURE APPLICATIONS
Addictions

The most common addictions are cravings for food, nicotine and alcohol, and dependence on drugs and narcotics. Everybody has a latent tendency to develop some sort of addiction, which may be bound up with repressed aggression needing a substitute outlet.

Ear acupuncture is well known as an effective treatment for addictions, but for best results you need to have two or three courses of the 'addiction programme' with an experienced acupuncturist. Combined with ear acupressure, this should prevent a relapse. People with milder forms of addiction should be able to achieve long-lasting results from acupressure alone.

What are the symptoms?

The over-riding element is an unhealthy craving for food, cigarettes, alcohol, or certain drugs. Very few people manage to overcome it by willpower alone, and the longer it goes on, the more difficult it is to stop.

What are the causes?

In some cases, the body becomes dependent on the substance to which it is addicted. When this substance is withdrawn, the body suffers withdrawal symptoms which vary according to the type of addiction involved. Acupressure helps the addict through this stage by retarding the body's reactions. In other cases, the dependence on the substance and the craving for it are psychological. Whatever the cause, apply acupressure to the appropriate points described below.

Body acupressure

The psychological relief point is the *tsu-san-li*, on the lower leg, directly beneath the tip of the ring finger when the palm of the hand is placed on the kneecap. Massage it downwards. Next, the *chin-wei* point at the base of the breastbone should be massaged upwards, and you should combine this with the *hon-ting*, which should be

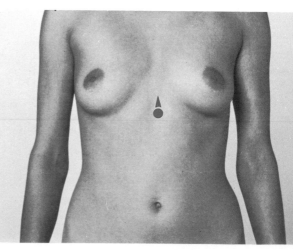

massaged forwards. This point lies in a small hollow, in the centre of the skull, two and a half to three finger-widths behind an imaginary line between the ears. Body acupressure in this case is less effective than ear acupressure.

Ear acupressure

There are two key points on the right ear, at the top and bottom of the lobe, towards the front. These should be massaged downwards. There is also a whole row of important points on the back edge of the ear, which should be massaged upwards. It is a good idea to put one of the fingers of your other hand behind your ear in this case, so that you can apply this massage accurately.

On the left ear, you need only massage the central energy point – on the ridge where it emerges from the central hollow – in a backwards and downwards direction. The other point, just in front of the top of the lobe, should be massaged downwards.

Treatment

During the acute stage of withdrawal, apply ear acupressure from two to five times a day, for five minutes at a time. After this, you can change to alternate days of ear and body acupressure. To prevent a return to the addiction, you should continue with acupressure once or twice a week for three to five months.

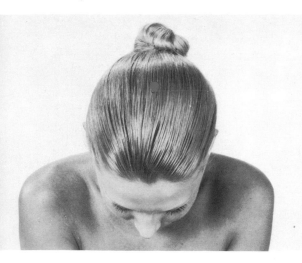

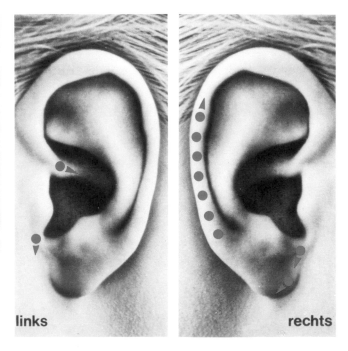

links   rechts

23

Anxiety

We are always reading nowadays about students' anxiety over examinations, and the stresses to which even schoolchildren are subjected in our competitive society. A great many adults suffer from anxiety too: for example, employees who are afraid of losing their jobs or housewives who feel incapable of looking after their children properly, or of fulfilling their role of wife, mother, cook, and companion, and of having a stabilizing influence on the whole family. One result of all this is that the consumption of tranquillizers is now running at the rate of tons and tons each year.

What are the symptoms?

At first the illness is scarcely noticed because, with the exception of examination stress, it starts subconsciously. Afterwards, it develops rapidly, revealing itself in a variety of ways. The housewife, for example, may be afraid to cross the road, while a manager may shut himself away in his office for fear of saying the wrong thing and at night may suffer from nightmares. Schoolchildren or students approaching an exam may find themselves incapable of bringing out a single word even though they are thoroughly on top of the subject.

What are the causes?

Stress of this kind is often due to a lack of self-confidence, caused by some failure in upbringing or excessive parental expectations centred on some ideal. Less often, over-anxiety is part of a hereditary disease; in these cases clarification from a doctor should be sought.

Body acupressure

The point 'heavenly calm' (in Chinese, *tsu-san-li*) should be massaged downwards. This point lies immediately below the tip of the ring finger when the palm of the hand is placed on the kneecap. Another important point acts as a stimulus on the psyche and the heart (in Chinese, *shao-chong*). This is situated on the inside of the last joint of the little finger and should be massaged across the back of the finger, below the nail, from the inside out.

You should also massage another point, about two finger-widths below and the same

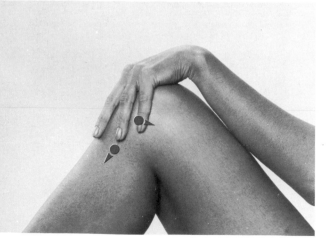

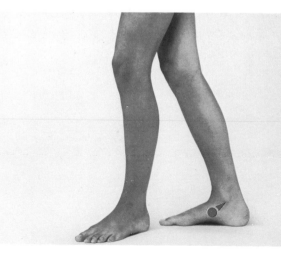

distance in front of the inner anklebone. It lies in a little hollow, called 'valley of light' (in Chinese, *jan-ku*). Massage it towards the anklebone itself. Finally, there is the 'energy-balancing' point (in Chinese, *chin-wei*) situated at the lowest tip of the breastbone. Massage it upwards.

Ear acupressure

There are two important points on the right ear. The first, near the front of the lobe, should be massaged upwards: the second, at the edge of the triangular-shaped hollow near the top of the ear, should be massaged towards the front. Reverse the directions for the left ear.

Treatment

Ear acupressure and body acupressure should be carried out on alternate days for about five minutes a day. If examination stress is likely, start acupressure a week or two before the exam takes place.

Patients on tranquillizers, once they begin to feel better as a result of acupressure, should be able to reduce their drug intake slowly, and in proportion to their improvement, but only in consultation with their doctor. They often find that they can give them up completely.

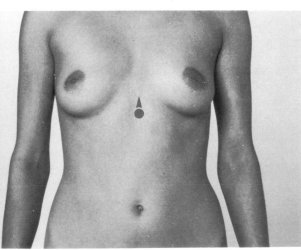

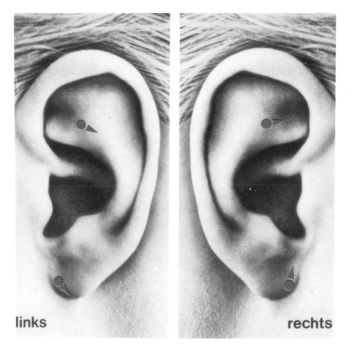

links   rechts

25

Appetite

Loss of appetite in children is usually only a passing phase and many a former 'faddy eater' turns out to be a well-built individual who can look back in amusement at the skinny creature he once used to be. Occasionally, however, this condition can give cause for concern. A seriously underweight child may even be at risk if he lacks the reserves of strength necessary to fight off an infectious disease, such as influenza or pneumonia.

What are the symptoms?

Children often eat poorly because they don't like what is put in front of them, or because they are daydreaming. But if they toy with their favourite food, or leave it untouched, and their body weight is 15–20 per cent below normal, something must be done about it.

What are the causes?

Sometimes loss of appetite is connected with physical development but it may also be the first sign of a serious problem. If you suspect this to be the case, go to your doctor straightaway. If, for example, an infectious disease is about to strike, the application of acupressure, in con-sultation with your doctor, may reduce the strain on the patient's reserves of energy. Loss of appetite, particularly in girls, may be due to psychological causes, and can assume strange forms. In such cases, acupressure should only be practised in collaboration with a psycho-therapist.

Body acupressure

The main point is the 'inner barrier' (in Chinese, *nei-kuan*), two or three finger-widths below the base of the palm, in the middle of the inside lower arm. Massage this towards the hand. If the problem is more psychologically based, use the stimulus point for the psyche and the heart, *shao-chong*, on the inside of the last joint of the little finger. Massage this across the back of the finger, below the nail, from the inside out.

There is also the stimulus point for the functions of the stomach (in Chinese, *chieh-hsi*), which is situated in the middle, and at the front, of the ankle joint. Massage it towards the toes. It is also worth while to apply acupressure to the 'centre of the stomach' point (in Chinese, *chung-kuan*), midway between the navel and the lower end of the breastbone. Massage it upwards.

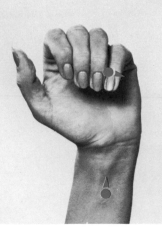

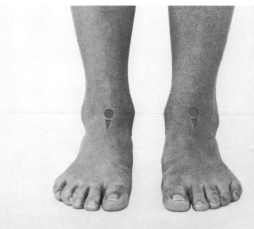

Ear acupressure

Two points should be treated. The first lies close to the back of the lobe and the point on the right ear should be massaged upwards and backwards. The second is the point of the solar plexus, the abdominal nerve centre. It will be found at the beginning of the central ridge and should be massaged upwards and forwards, along the ridge itself. The points on the left ear are the same but the directions of massage should be reversed.

Treatment

Carry out body acupressure and ear acupressure on alternate days, for two to three minutes at a time, about a quarter of an hour before meals. It does not matter whether you begin with body acupressure or ear acupressure. In the case of small children, the parents should carry out the massage to start with, but if possible the child should learn the technique so that he can massage the points himself later on.

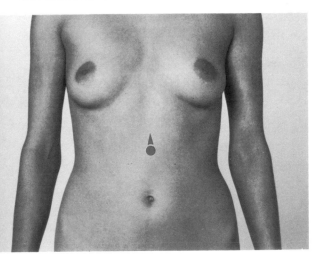

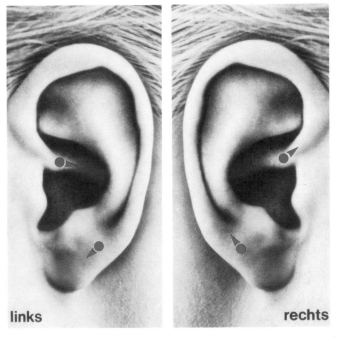

links　　　　rechts

Arm and shoulder pains

Pain and immobility in these parts is very common. Usually, your doctor will recommend an X-ray to make sure that no bones are broken, but even then the pain may persist for some time and be too deep-seated to respond to normal treatment. In such cases start acupressure as soon as possible.

What are the symptoms?

The pain is worst at night. It is not necessarily in one place but in different places in turn. Some of the strength in the affected arm is lost, due to the fact that you cannot move it without pain.

What are the causes?

As a rule, these pains are the result of a fall on the shoulder but they may also be due to some other form of injury such as a strain, a jolt or heavy blow, or an accident.

Body acupressure

The point the Chinese call the *ta-chui*, just below the prominent seventh cervical vertebra, should be massaged firmly upwards. The key point for the arms, the *t'ien-chaio*, lies halfway along an imaginary line between the previous point and the highest part of the shoulder. It is not a difficult point to find, being particularly sensitive to pressure. Massage it in the direction of the ear. The *chien-yu* (shoulderbone) point lies on the front outer part of the shoulders, in a little hollow which you can feel when you bend your arm upwards. This point should be massaged towards the neck.

A point with a more local effect is the *pi-hao* (arm-muscle), on the outside of the upper arm, just below the base of the triangular shoulder muscle. (If you raise your arm to the side you can see this deltoid muscle quite clearly.) Massage it upwards. The *san-li* point lies three to four finger-widths from the crease of the elbow when the arm is bent, on an imaginary line towards the thumb. Massage it upwards.

There are two more general points: the first, the *ho-ku*, is two finger-widths below the centre of the index finger knuckle, and half a finger-width towards the thumb. The second, the *wan-ku*, is on the outside edge of the wrist, in a small hollow. Massage both these points in the direction of the elbow.

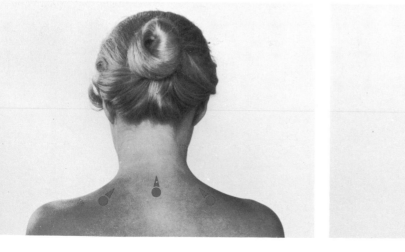

Ear acupressure

The points for arm and shoulder pains are situated midway between the back edge of the ear and the central hollow, and should be massaged firmly upwards. The equivalent points behind the ear, in the hollow but slightly nearer the edge, should also be massaged upwards. These are important for helping movement of the arms and shoulders. An exception to the rule in this case is that both ears should be massaged in the same direction.

Treatment

Ear and body acupressure should be alternated daily, one to three times a day, for periods of five to ten minutes, depending on the severity of the complaint. If your doctor confirms that you also have some form of spinal injury, you should apply the appropriate acupressure treatment for that too (see page 138).

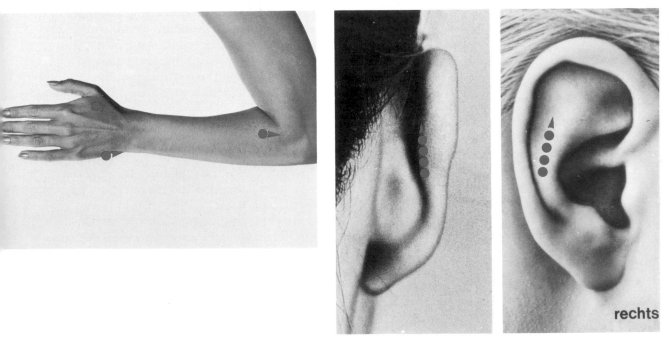

rechts

29

Bedwetting

Bedwetting puts parents in a dilemma, as scolding does not help, and no one wants to give pills to a small child. Acupressure can help here, too.

Though rare, the complaint can also occur in adults, when it is a sign of an approaching nervous complaint or a deep emotional upset. In this case consultation with a doctor is necessary.

What are the symptoms?

Although the child is beyond the nappy stage, he wets the bed at night, and sometimes wets himself during the day. The same treatment applies in both cases.

What are the causes?

Usually, bedwetting is due to a psychological and functional weakness of the bladder. The psychological disturbance may be due to a lack of harmony in the home, while in school-children it may be caused by competitive stress. It can also be due to dreams occurring in deep sleep in an over-imaginative child.

The patient should first be medically examined, so as to exclude any possibility of chronic inflammation or organic disturbance of the bladder. The doctor will usually diagnose a functional bladder weakness.

Body acupressure

Massage in a forward direction the *pai-hui* point, which lies in the centre of the skull at the top of an imaginary line connecting both ears. Next, the *san-yin-chiao* point, four to five of the child's (not your own) finger-widths above the inner point of the anklebone, at the rear edge of the shinbone, should be massaged upwards.

Another point requiring treatment is the 'heavenly calm' (in Chinese, *tsu-san-li*), which lies immediately below the tip of the ring finger when the child places his palm on his kneecap. Massage it downwards. Next comes the stimulus point for the functions of the bladder (in Chinese, *chih-yin*), near the outside of the last joint of the little toe. Massage the back of the toe, just below the nail, from the outside in. Be careful not to press too hard, otherwise it may be painful.

There is one other point (not shown) which can be treated, the *chung-chi*, as it is known in

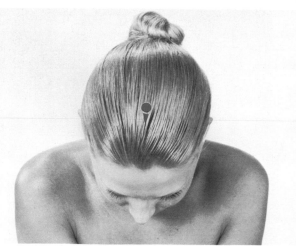

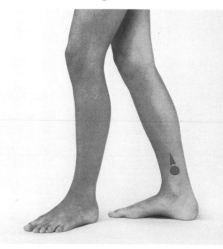

China. This lies on an imaginary line between the navel and the bladder, just above the latter, and is generally sensitive to acupressure in an upward direction. It is called the 'alarm point', and is the energy point for the bladder.

Ear acupressure

There are two points on the ear which need treatment. On the right ear, the bladder point which lies in the upper hollow is massaged forwards, while the psychological relief point, at the front of the outer ridge, should be massaged upwards. Massage the same points in the opposite directions on the left ear.

Treatment

As usual, ear acupressure and body acupressure should be alternated daily for five to ten minutes at a time, just before bedtime. If the child has been put on sedatives or antidepressants by the doctor, you should, in consultation with him, be able to reduce the dosage gradually until they are no longer required. Teach the child to massage himself, but make sure that the treatment is properly carried out.

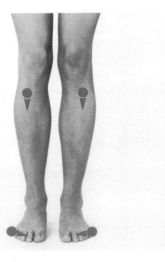

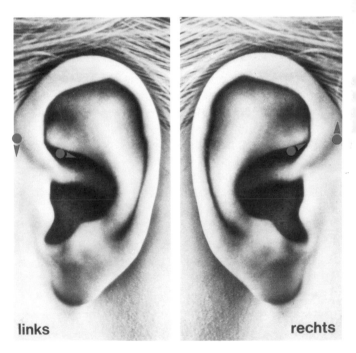

links   rechts

Belching and swallowing air

There is always a certain amount of air in the stomach. Belching brings up the air which is swallowed when eating and drinking. Small babies burp naturally during and after feeding, and do not need acupressure unless the activity is prolonged.

What are the symptoms?

Swallowing air is often followed by belching, accompanied by a sour taste in the mouth, and can be very unpleasant. There is also the possibility of hiccups and, in extreme cases, vomiting.

What is the cause?

The most common cause is extreme nervousness or nervous tension. In chronic cases it may be due to organic problems requiring medical treatment. You can relieve or overcome the symptoms by the techniques explained here, but this is only a part of the treatment. It is, if anything, more important to deal with the root cause of the problem, and appropriate advice will be found in the section headed 'Nervousness and Irritability' (page 114).

Body acupressure

Massage should be applied, in an upward direction, to the 'centre of the stomach' point (in Chinese, *chung-kuan*), midway between the navel and the lower point of the breastbone, and two other points, the *shang-kuan* and the *chü-ch'üch*, lying just above it.

Belching is helped by treating the point at the top of the breastbone (at the level of the first rib), called *hsüan-chi* in Chinese. Massage it upwards. In order to regulate the functioning of the body's waste disposal system, it is helpful to massage the appropriate point, *chieh-hsi*, in the middle and at the front of the ankle joint. Massage it towards the toes.

In persistent cases it may be necessary to massage further points on the back, which will require outside help. These are the 'point of equilibrium' of the diaphragm (in Chinese, *ko-shu*), two to three finger-widths to the side of the lower edge of the seventh thoracic vertebra,

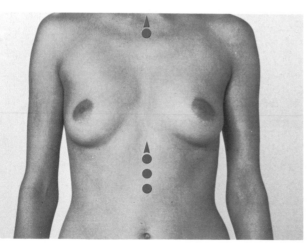

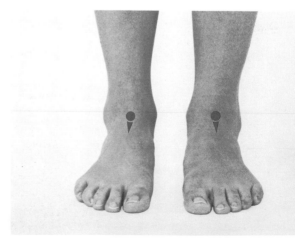

and the 'point of equilibrium' of the stomach (in Chinese, *wei-shu*) two to three finger-widths to the side of the lower edge of the twelfth thoracic vertrebra. Massage both points downwards.

Ear acupressure

Apply acupressure to the point of the solar plexus on the right ear. This is a nerve centre which was formerly also known as the 'brain of the abdomen'. It is situated at the beginning of the central ridge of the ear, and should be massaged along the ridge, upwards and forwards. Behind the right ear lies the point of the throat, on the edge of the hollow. This should be massaged upwards. The left ear need not usually be treated.

Treatment

For normal – that is, infrequent – hiccuping, it is usually sufficient to apply a good bout of massage to the point of the solar plexus on the ear. In severe cases of swallowing air and belching, however, it is advisable to consult the psychotherapist and, with his consent, to apply body and ear acupressure on alternate days to the points described above, and to the points related to nervousness (see page 114).

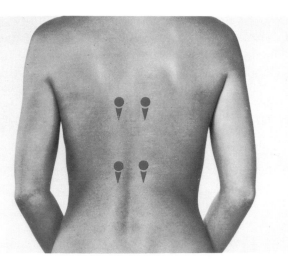

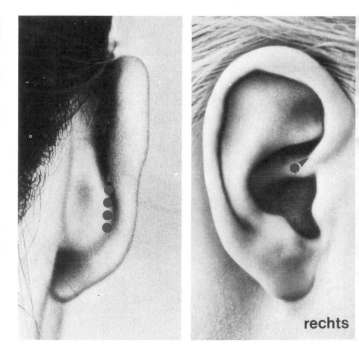

rechts

33

Bladder disorders

1 Inflammation

Cystitis is the most common complaint of the bladder, usually developing from an apparently harmless chill on the stomach into a severe inflammation. It is common in young women, because they tend to wear thin under-clothes. Keep your stomach warm if you want to avoid inflammation of the bladder.

What are the symptoms?

Passing water produces a pronounced burning sensation, and the patient urinates more often than usual.

What is the cause?

Exposure to severe cold is the usual cause of a stomach chill, which may then develop into chronic cystitis. This, in turn, may lead to inflammation of the kidneys (nephritis). In other words, what starts off as a harmless complaint can become a serious illness. In such cases, you should see your doctor immediately. He will usually prescribe drugs to reduce the inflam-

mation and, in consultation with him, you can apply acupressure with a view to curing the cystitis more rapidly, as well as preventing it from developing into a chronic condition and avoiding a relapse once it has been cured.

Body acupressure

The Chinese point for strengthening the bladder, the *chih-yin*, lies next to the outside edge of the last joint of the little toe: massage it from the outside in. The *san-yin-chiao* point, four finger-widths above the inner point of the anklebone, at the back of the shinbone, should be massaged upwards.

The energy points for the bladder are the *chung-chi*, just above the bladder in the centre of the lower abdomen, and the *ch'i-hai*, two to three (on fat people, four to five) finger-widths below the navel. Massage both upwards.

In cases of prolonged, chronic illness, outside help should be sought to massage the 'point of equilibrium' of the bladder, the *p'ang kuang shu*, which is situated at the side of and level

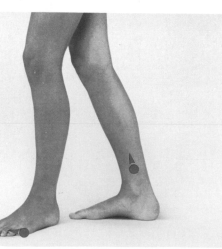
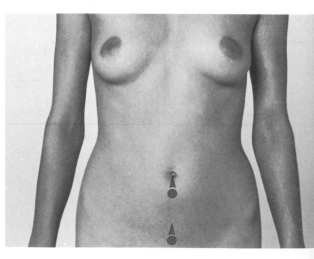

with the top of the crease dividing the buttocks. This point is very sensitive to pressure and is not difficult to find.

Ear acupressure

Apply treatment to the bladder point, in the upper ridge of the right ear, and the general energy point, the nerve centre of the solar plexus, at the point where the ridge emerges from the central hollow. Massage both upwards and forwards. The same points can also be massaged on the left ear, but in the opposite direction.

Treatment

Apply ear acupressure and body acupressure on alternate days. Generally speaking, treatment lasting five to ten minutes once a day is enough to begin with. Later, as a preventative measure, this can be reduced to once or twice a week. Make sure you wear warm underclothes, and avoid sitting on cold surfaces.

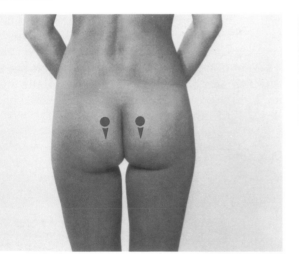

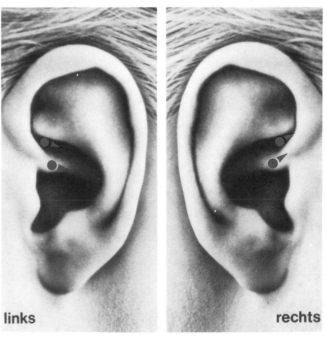

links   rechts

Bladder disorders

2 Over-active bladder

This means excessive urination for no organic reason. It is an unpleasant disorder which plagues nervous people, and is especially common among women.

What are the symptoms?

Sufferers find it necessary to go to the lavatory as many as twenty times a day, and then find that they pass very little water in relation to the need – sometimes only a few drops.

What is the cause?

It often begins as a harmless stomach chill (in which case the acupressure treatment described in the previous section can be applied), but even when the inflammation is completely cleared up, and the doctor gives the patient a clean bill of health following a urine test, there is a persistent, nervous need to urinate which cannot be overcome by willpower. Before beginning acupressure, you should get your doctor to confirm that the disorder is not due to chronic inflammation of the kidneys or bladder.

Body acupressure

Apply treatment to the *pai-hui* point on the top of the skull, in the centre of an imaginary line between the ears: massage it forwards. Next, the two energy points for the bladder, the *chung-chi* and the *ch'i-hai*, the first in the middle of the lower abdomen immediately above the bladder, and the second two to three finger-widths (on fat people four to five) below the navel, should be massaged upwards.

For relief of tension, massage the *tsu-san-li* point downwards. This is also known as 'asiatic peace', and is on the side of the leg, at a point below the ring finger when the palm of the hand is placed on the kneecap. Another point giving relief is the *t'ai-ch'ung*, which is a good two finger-widths above the crease between the first and second toes; this should be massaged towards the ankle.

Ear acupressure

The point of the bladder, which on the right ear lies at the front of the hollow, should be

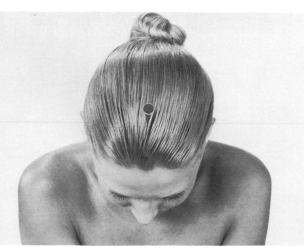

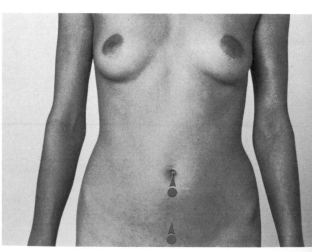

massaged forwards, and the psychological relief point, where the ear joins the head, should be massaged upwards. There is also a central nervous point, which is linked to the thought area of the brain, and which lies at the front of the lobe: massage it upwards. As shown in the illustration, the points on the left ear should be massaged in the opposite direction to those on the right ear.

Treatment

Ear acupressure and body acupressure should be alternated daily. In the case of a severe onset, apply treatment for five to ten minutes twice a day, reducing to once a day, then once a week, as the patient's condition improves. During the period of treatment, strong food and drink should be avoided.

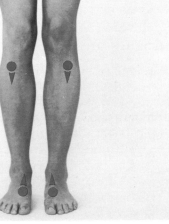

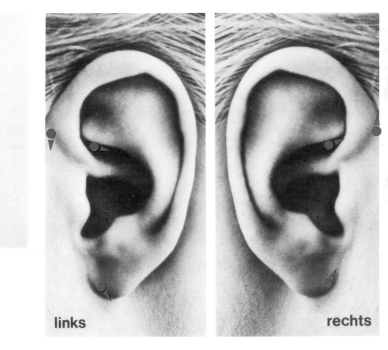

links   rechts

Circulation disorders of the arms and hands

Complaints about cold hands and feet (see page 42) are commonplace. If you suffer from both, you should combine the two treatments by applying both forms of ear acupressure on one day, and both forms of body acupressure on the next, and so on. Smoking contributes to circulation problems, so you should cut down, or better still give up smoking altogether (see page 22 for acupressure treatment for addictions).

What are the symptoms?

First you have cold fingers, then cold hands: sometimes even your arms get cold as well, but this is rare.

What are the causes?

In simple terms, the vessels carrying your blood are too narrow for the task, with the result that too little fresh (arterial) blood reaches your hands. The constriction may be due to the state of your nerves, and in this case acupressure gives excellent relief. Another cause is the build-up of calcium salts on the linings of the arteries. If this has reached an advanced state, acupressure cannot help. Or there may be a combination of causes.

You should consult your doctor for an examination and advice. Usually he will prescribe drugs to improve your circulation. Combine these with acupressure, in consultation with your doctor.

Body acupressure

The first point is the *chung-ch'ung*, which is the stimulus point for the circulation. It lies near the lower corner of the middle fingernail, on the index finger side, and should be massaged across the finger, below the nail, towards the ring finger. If you have high blood pressure, massage this point very gently. Another important point is the *hou-hsi*, on the side of the hand, just below the knuckle joint of the little finger. Massage it towards the elbow.

Next comes the *ho-ku* point, two finger-widths below the knuckle of the index finger

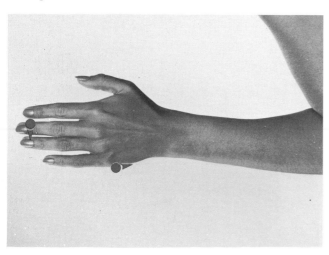

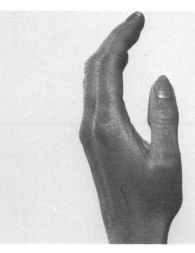

and half a finger-width towards the thumb. Massage this towards the elbow; likewise the *san-li* point, which lies two to three finger-widths in front of the crease which forms at your elbow when you bend your arm. At the very end of this same crease there is the stimulus point, *ch'üh-ch'ih*, which can be massaged upwards if required.

Ear acupressure

Massage both ears, even though one hand may seem to be colder than the other. There are several points for the arms and hands, all situated between the central hollow and the outer edge, most of them on a central line.

Massage them all in an upward direction. Also treat the general energy point, on the ridge where it emerges from the central hollow: massage forwards and upwards. On the left ear, all the directions of massage should be reversed, as shown.

Treatment

Ear and body acupressure should be alternated daily, one to three times a day, for five to ten minutes, depending on the severity of the case. If your doctor has prescribed drugs to improve your circulation, continue to take them, and apply the acupressure treatment at the same time.

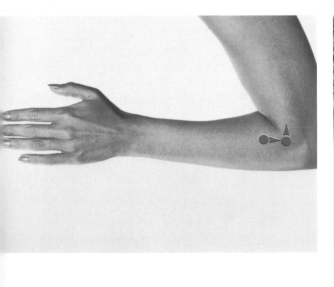

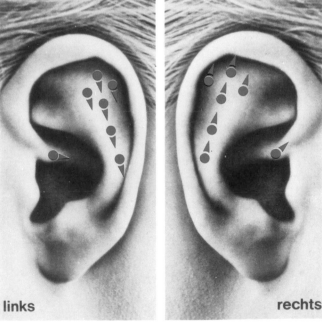

links **rechts**

39

Circulation disorders of the brain

Our life expectancy has been extended over the years; the average for women is seventy years, for men slightly less. While this may generally be a good thing, old age also brings its problems, the most common of which is poor circulation. Elderly people frequently suffer from poor circulation to the brain.

What are the symptoms?

The first and most obvious signs are forgetfulness and loss of concentration, but there are others which may take the form of giddiness or trembling. If the circulation is very poor, the patient may behave irrationally or even suffer a personality change, to the extent that a quiet person will suddenly become angry and aggressive, and vice-versa. As a rule, this type of patient is put into an old people's home.

What are the causes?

There are two. First, there is the weakening of the heart which comes with old age and second,

there is an increasing thickening of the arteries, due to calcium deposits which restrict the flow of fresh blood to the brain. Any agitation affecting the so-called sympathetic nerves will also contribute to the narrowing of the arteries. If the cause is purely one of calcium deposits in the arteries, acupressure cannot help. However, if the problem is mainly one of nerves, there is a good chance of its being successful, but make sure you carry out the treatment in consultation with your doctor.

Body acupressure

The principal Chinese point is the *pai-hui*, which is in the centre of the skull, on an imaginary line between the ears. This is surrounded by four other points ('wisdom of four gods'), one and a half to two finger-widths to the front, back, and each side of the previous point. Massage all five points towards the forehead.

The general energy point, the *ch'i-hai* ('sea of energy'), which lies two to three (on fat people,

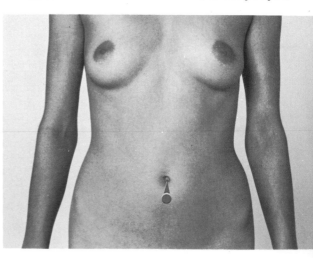

four to five) finger-widths below the navel, should be massaged upwards.

If you have low blood pressure, acupressure of the *chung-ch'ung* point, which stimulates the circulation, is especially beneficial. This lies near the corner at the base of the middle fingernail, on the side nearest the index finger, and the finger should be massaged below the nail, towards the ring finger. If you have high blood pressure, massage this last point very gently.

Ear acupressure

The reflex points for the brain and its blood supply are all on the lobe. On the right ear,

massage them upwards and backwards, and on the left ear downwards and forwards. Also massage the area at the front of the ear, from bottom to top on the right ear, and vice-versa on the left.

Treatment

Ear and body acupressure should be alternated daily, one to three times a day for five to ten minutes at a time, depending on the severity of the complaint. Any drugs prescribed should be taken in combination with acupressure treatment. If you smoke, make up your mind to give it up (see the section on addictions, page 22).

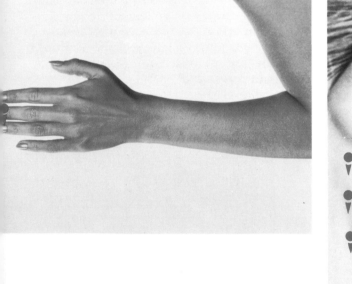

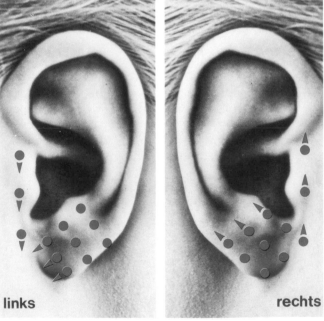

links   rechts

41

Circulation of the feet and legs

This complaint is sometimes called 'smoker's leg' or 'shopwindow disease' because a person who starts to feel sharp pains in the calves of his or her legs and has to stop walking may look in the nearest shopwindow so as not to appear conspicuous!

What are the symptoms?

At first you notice that you have perpetually cold feet; later, your lower legs feel cold and your skin turns a mottled, brown colour where the tissue is starting to die.

What are the causes?

The vessels carrying the blood to the feet are either too narrow or they have become congested, so that insufficient fresh (arterial) blood reaches the feet. Narrow veins may be due to the state of your 'sympathetic' nerves, in which case acupressure can give satisfactory relief, but if the pain is caused by calcium deposits on the linings of the arteries, or a blood clot, acupressure cannot help. Your doctor will be able to isolate the cause, and will almost certainly prescribe drugs to improve your circulation. Combine these with acupressure, in consultation with your doctor.

Body acupressure

The first point is the *san-yin-chiao*, four to five finger-widths above the inner anklebone, and this should be massaged upwards. If the skin in this area is in a poor condition, apply the massage very gently.

There is another point, the *tsu-san-li* ('heavenly healer of the feet and knees'), which lies directly beneath the tip of the ring finger when the palm of the hand is placed on the kneecap. Massage it downwards.

It is important to massage the *yang-ling-ch'uan* point, immediately forward and down from the top of the outer legbone (fibula); massage it downwards.

The general stimulus point for the circulation, the *chung-ch'ung*, is near the lower corner

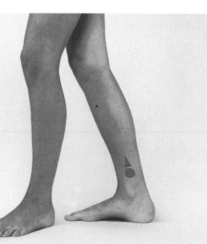

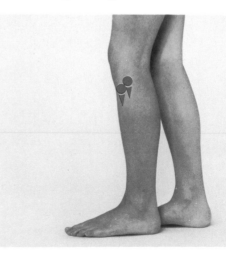

of the middle fingernail, on the index finger side. Massage the finger, just below the nail, towards the ring finger. If you have high blood pressure, massage this last point very gently.

Ear acupressure

Massage the points on both ears, even though one foot may seem colder than the other. The points associated with the feet are in the upper, triangular hollow, towards the front of the ear. On the right ear these should all be massaged forwards and upwards. The general energy point, on the ridge where it emerges from the central hollow, should also be massaged forwards and upwards. Reverse the directions on the left ear, as shown.

Treatment

Ear and body acupressure should be alternated daily, one to three times a day, for five to ten minutes at a time, depending on the severity of the case. Any drugs prescribed should be taken in combination with the acupressure treatment. If you smoke, you should make every effort to give it up (see the section on addictions, page 22).

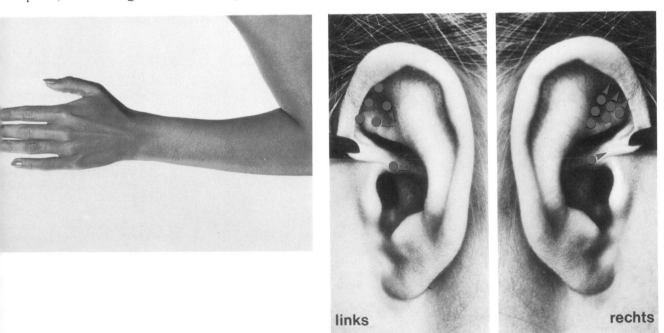

links   rechts

Colds and catarrh

Inflammation of the mucous membrane of the nose, which you get with the common cold, can, in severe cases, lead to inflammation of the sinuses. These are cavities in the hollow bones surrounding the nose, which communicate with it by openings in the sidewall. In certain circumstances these openings swell up, causing pressure and pain in the cavities. This requires treatment by an E.N.T. (ear, nose and throat) specialist, who will prescribe treatment to re-open the cavities and dissipate the secretion. However, if you apply acupressure as soon as the trouble starts, it should not get to this stage.

What are the symptoms?

We all know what it is like to have a red, runny nose. If the sinuses are also inflamed, you will notice some discomfort if you tap the area around the nose lightly with your finger. An X-ray will confirm the complaint.

What is the cause?

Most colds occur with the start of the cold, damp season. If you have a bad bout, and also lack resistance, the sinuses may become inflamed too. Cold feet, especially if they are wet, often bring on colds, which may be explained by the old Chinese theory of acupuncture. This says that the bladder and stomach meridians begin at the feet, then spread upwards over the whole body, ending at the nose and sinuses. The stimulus point for both meridians is in the foot, so wearing warm socks or stockings and sensible shoes when the weather is bad has a beneficial effect on them. If the cold has already started, acupressure will bring relief, but if the sinuses are inflamed, see your E.N.T. specialist.

Body acupressure

The first two points are the *chü-chiao*, which is level with the outer edge of the nostril and about one and a half finger-widths to the side (directly below the pupil), and the *szu-pai*, which is a little hollow two finger-widths below the pupil. Massage both points downwards.

Next, the points *ying-hsiang* and *ho-chiao* should be massaged upwards. The first of these is at the top end of the crease, which runs from the side of the nose to the outside of the mouth,

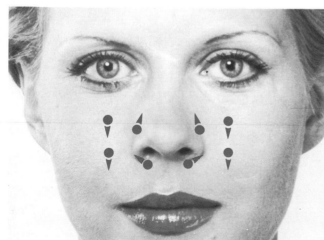
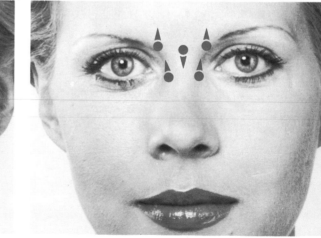

while the second is one and a half finger-widths lower down.

The *inn-trang* point, which is at the very top of the nose, midway between the eyebrows, should be massaged downwards. The points *ching-ming* and *ts'uan-chu*, on the other hand, should be massaged upwards. These are situated close to each other, the first on each side of the bridge, the second at the beginning of each eyebrow.

An important point for the membranes is the *ho-ki*, on the back of the hand, two finger-widths below the knuckle of the index finger and half a finger-width towards the thumb. Massage it in the direction of the elbow.

Ear acupressure

The points for the nose and sinuses, on the right ear lobe, should be massaged upwards, or upwards and backwards, as shown. The central energy point, on the ridge, where it emerges from the central hollow, should be massaged forwards and upwards. On the left ear, massage in the opposite directions.

Treatment

Ear and body acupressure should be alternated daily, one to three times a day, for five to ten minutes, depending on the severity of the complaint. Remember to wear warm socks or stockings and sensible shoes, and do not give up any medicine you may have had prescribed without consulting your doctor first.

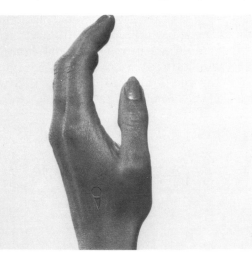

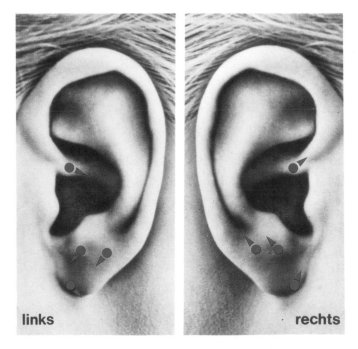

links　　　　　**rechts**

45

Constipation

1 Constipation due to intestinal sluggishness

As a rule, you should have one bowel action a day, but two a day, or one every other day, is perfectly normal. There are two kinds of constipation. In the first case, the intestine gets sluggish and out of condition, and is unable to expel its contents. In the second case, which occurs in nervous people, the intestine is subjected to tension and prevented from functioning properly. I will deal with the first kind here, and the second on the following pages.

What are the symptoms?

You find that a bowel action is protracted and difficult, and only occurs every few days, with the result that the stools are dry and hard. Severe constipation causes the stomach to stretch painfully. You may also suffer from a loss of appetite, an unpleasant taste in the mouth and bad breath, a furred tongue, headaches, or general lassitude. As a rule, all these symptoms disappear soon after a bowel action has occurred.

What are the causes?

If there is too little roughage in your diet, most of your food is digested in the area of the small intestine, and what residue there is stays in the large intestine and thickens more than it should. This in turn affects the muscles which have the function of expelling the contents of the intestine. Many foods and medicines contribute towards constipation, as well as lack of exercise and bad toilet training. You should try to train yourself to open your bowels once a day, at about the same time if possible.

There are other causes of constipation, such as intestinal tumours in the elderly, but in these cases a thorough medical examination is essential.

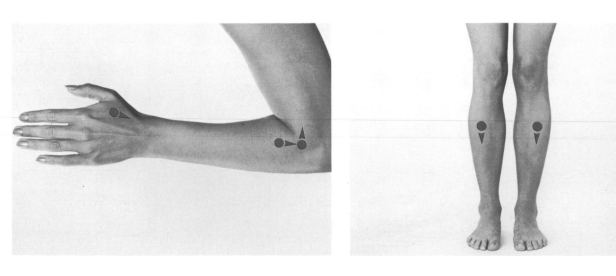

Body acupressure

The Chinese points for the functions of the large intestine, which are on the hand and arm, are all important and should be massaged, in turn, in an upward direction. They are the *ho-ku*, the *san-li* and the stimulus point, *ch-üh-ch'ih*. The first is two finger-widths below the knuckle of the index finger and half a finger-width towards the thumb, the third is at the outer end of the elbow crease (when the arm is bent), and the second is three to four finger-widths below the previous point, on a direct line between points one and three.

Another effective point is the *chü-shü shang-lien*, eight finger-widths below the centre of the kneecap and two finger-widths towards the outside of the leg. Massage it firmly downwards. Finally, there is the 'point of equilibrium' of the large intestine, the *ta-ch'ang-shu*, which is two to three finger-widths to the side of the base of the fourth lumbar vertebra: massage it downwards.

Ear acupressure

Treatment occurs mainly on the left ear and, as 'motor-points' are used, they are all behind the ear. Those for the large intestine lie at the top of the main hollow, near the head, and should be massaged firmly upwards. On the right ear, the points shown should also be massaged upwards, particularly if stimulation of the small intestine is also desired.

Treatment

Ear and body acupressure should be alternated daily, one to three times a day, for five to ten minutes, depending on the severity of the condition. Make sure you take plenty of roughage in your diet and try to develop 'regular' habits. You will gradually be able to reduce your intake of laxatives.

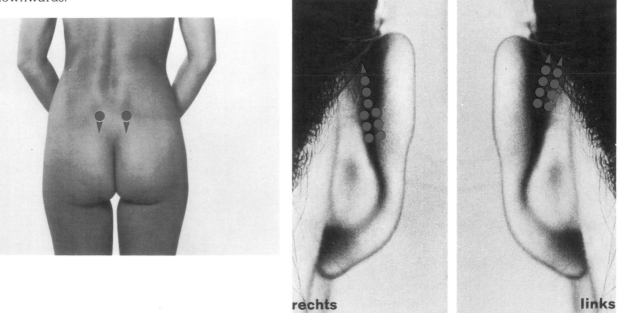

rechts   links

47

Constipation

2 Constipation due to a spastic colon (intestinal cramp)

Constipation due to intestinal cramp is usually a sign of nervousness and is common among people of an unstable disposition. It also shows itself in other disorders of the stomach and small intestine. In this case, the stools are small and pellet-like or compressed together, reminiscent of sheep's droppings.

What are the symptoms?

Cramps, which are brought on by tension in the intestine, cause the latter to contract in places and thereby hinder a bowel action. In turn this leads to an unpleasant 'overfull' feeling, 'tugging' pains in the stomach and often colic pains as well.

What are the causes?

Tension in the intestine is rooted in the excessive nervousness of the patient, which in turn is conditioned by psychological factors, so this complaint should be regarded as a psychosomatic illness. It should be left to a specialist doctor, psychiatrist or psychotherapist to determine the fundamental cause of the abnormal tension and nervousness. A course of acupressure, carried out in consultation with the doctor, will give excellent results.

Body acupressure

The principal point is the *ho-ku* which, according to the Chinese, has a 'harmonizing' effect on the large intestine. It lies two finger-widths below the knuckle of the index finger and half a finger-width towards the thumb, and should be massaged in the direction of the elbow. The *hou-hsi* point, in a small hollow just outside and below the little finger knuckle joint, should also be massaged towards the elbow.

Two other important points for the relief of tension are the *hsing-chien*, in the crease between the big toe and second toe, slightly nearer the big toe, and the *t'ai-chung*, two to three finger-widths higher up; massage both points firmly, towards the ankle.

The key point for psychological relief is the

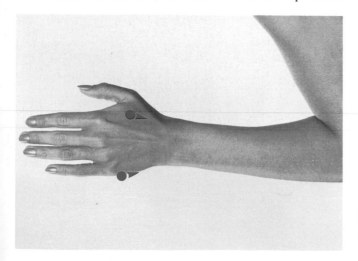

tsu-san-li, on the lower leg, directly beneath the tip of the ring finger when the palm of the hand is placed on the kneecap. Massage it downwards.

Ear acupressure

On the right ear, the psychological relief point is in front of the ear, where it joins the head. Massage it firmly upwards; likewise the point at the top forward edge of the lobe. On the left ear, massage the same points in a downward direction. The points for the large intestine, in the hollow above the central ridge, should be massaged in a backward and downward direction on *both* ears.

Treatment

Ear and body acupressure should be alternated daily, for about ten minutes at a time, ideally half an hour before the hoped-for bowel action. If you are taking drugs for the relief of tension, you should gradually reduce them in consultation with your doctor.

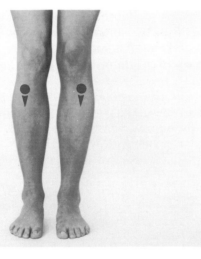

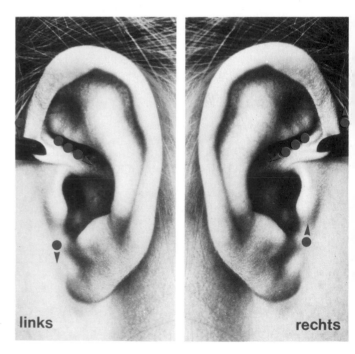

links   rechts

Coughs and bronchitis

Bronchitis, which is a very common complaint, due to ever-increasing air pollution and too much cigarette smoking, tends to be at its worst in spring and autumn. If you want to get rid of your smoker's cough you must first overcome the addiction by a course of anti-smoking treatment. Light smokers should be able to give up smoking by applying acupressure to themselves (see page 22). Others should visit an acupuncturist for treatment and then apply acupressure to prevent themselves taking up smoking again.

What are the symptoms?

It begins with occasional bouts of coughing, usually in the morning, and gradually gets chronic. In some cases your cough may be quite mild, more like a tickle in the back of the throat, while at the other extreme you can be racked by coughing, bringing up varying amounts of mucus at the same time.

What are the causes?

The root cause is irritation or inflammation in the air passages, starting above the lungs but later spreading down into them. Influenza can also develop into bronchitis. A very bad cough may be a sign of a malignant growth in the lung tissue. Whatever the cause, you should consult your doctor for an accurate diagnosis, then practise acupressure in consultation with him.

Body acupressure

The principal Chinese point is the *shu-fu*, on the lower edge of the collarbone, near the breastbone. Massage it upwards. Next, the two points, the *chin-wei* at the base of the breastbone, and the *tan-chung* ('centre of the breast') on the breastbone, level with a man's nipples, should be massaged upwards. The key point for all forms of congestion in the chest is the *lieh-ch'üeh*, two finger-widths above the palm of the hand, and this should be massaged towards the base of the thumb.

For chronic bronchitis you should also massage the *ta-chui* (big vertebra) point in an upward direction. As its name implies, this point lies immediately below the prominent seventh cervical vertebra.

Finally, if you are bringing up mucus when

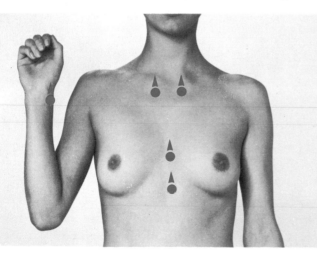
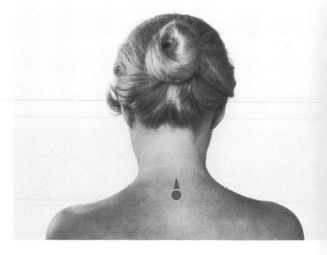

you cough, massage the *feng-lung* ('overfill') point. You can find it by taking the halfway point between the middle of the outer ankle-bone and the middle of the kneecap, and measuring one finger-width to the outside, and you will recognize it by its sensitivity to pressure. Massage it downwards.

Ear acupressure

On the right ear massage the point for the bronchial tubes and the lungs and to relieve an irritating cough, massage the point of psychological relief, at the front of the ear, where it joins the head. In both cases massage upwards. For chronic bronchitis massage the same points on the left ear as well, this time in a downward direction.

Treatment

There is no point in applying acupressure in this instance unless you have given up smoking first. Then, ear and body acupressure should be alternated daily, for five to ten minutes at a time. You will soon be breathing more easily and feel healthier generally.

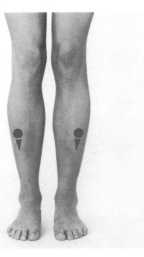

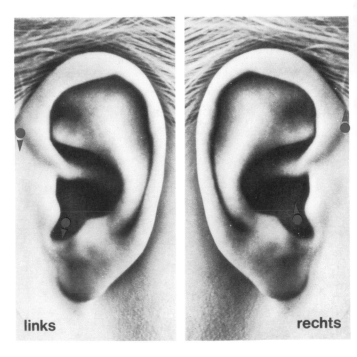

links   rechts

Depression

Nowadays, more and more people suffer from a feeling of despair and dejection. In fact, it is estimated that every third case of illness is due to so-called 'depression'. Loneliness or a disagreement with someone all too often leads to attempted suicide: in Britain alone there are about a hundred suicides a week.

What are the symptoms?

A true depression is, unfortunately, not easy to recognize at first, due to the fact that we all get a bit dejected and out-of-sorts at times, though these phases usually pass of their own accord. To make matters worse, the depression often hides behind other symptoms. For this reason we often speak of a 'hidden' depression, and a headache, a stomach upset, sleeplessness, or a 'heavy' feeling may be a sign of a hidden depression.

What are the causes?

There are two main kinds of depression. The first, which is hereditary, is called endogenous depression and does not respond to acupressure. The other kind is really a self-generated depression, the so-called exogenous form. It has been found that in depressed people the brain metabolism undergoes a change, and it is this disturbance which causes the depression. In a case of this sort, you should apply acupressure *only* in close consultation with your doctor.

Body acupressure

The principal Chinese point, which stimulates the heart and psyche, is the *shao-chong*, near the the inside lower corner of the little finger. This should be massaged across the finger below the nail, towards the outside edge. There is a second point called the *tung-li* ('link with the inner self'), one and a half to two finger-widths above the base of the palm, on a line with the little finger. Massage it towards the little finger.

If you are suffering from a marked lack of energy, massage the key energy point, the *ch'i-hai*, two or three (on fat people, four to five) finger-widths below the navel, in an upward direction. Another point, the *chin-wei*, at the base of the breastbone, should be massaged upwards.

The point which is especially beneficial in

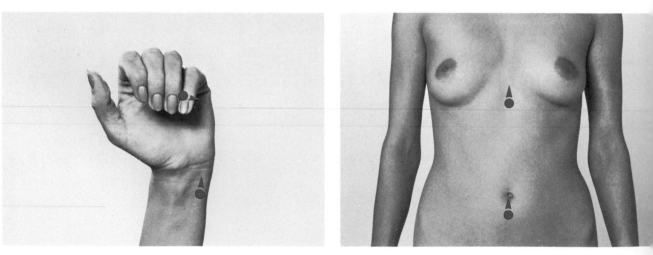

building up one's energy reserves is the *inn-po*, near the base of the big toenail on the inside of the foot, and this should be massaged towards the inner anklebone. For more restless forms of depression massage the *tsu-san-li* point. This is immediately beneath the tip of the ring finger when the palm of the hand is placed on the kneecap. Massage it downwards.

Ear acupressure

On the right ear, the key point for depression lies low down, towards the back of the lobe. Massage it upwards and backwards. For the nerve centre of the abdomen, massage the point on the central ridge, well towards the top. Also, the whole of the forward part of the ear should be massaged from bottom to top. There is one final point, on the edge of the upper, triangular hollow, and this should be massaged forwards. In severe cases of depression, massage the same points on the left ear as well, but in the opposite direction in each case.

Treatment

Don't give up if you fail to achieve overnight success, but keep on applying ear and body acupressure on alternate days, morning and evening, for five to ten minutes at a time. Also, keep on taking the drugs your doctor has prescribed (anti-depressants), until he says you can reduce your dosage.

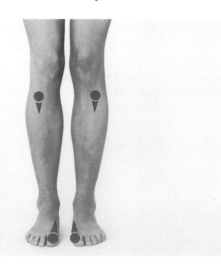

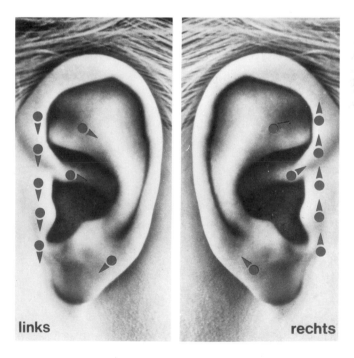

links   rechts

53

Diarrhoea

Diarrhoea, characterized by frequent bowel actions and the watery nature of the motions, is normally quite harmless. Acupressure helps to relieve the stomach cramps and the inflammation of the mucous membrane of the intestinal wall.

What are the symptoms?

Diarrhoea usually begins with a rumbling sensation in the intestines, followed by an urgent need to relieve the bowels. The motion itself is soft or runny or, in extreme cases, positively watery.

What are the causes?

The main causes are exposure to cold, extreme nervousness or too much eating and drinking of the wrong kind. Diarrohoea can also be caused by a virus infection, such as occurs from eating inadequately washed salads in hot countries, or from drinking impure water. In this case, your doctor will prescribe medicine to destroy the virus, and acupressure should be carried out in consultation with him.

Body acupressure

For the relief of stomach cramps the Chinese points *hsing-chien* and *t'ai-ch'ung* should be massaged. The first lies in the fold between the first and second toes (nearer the big toe), and the second about two finger-widths above. In both cases, massage the points towards the ankle.

The key point for diarrhoea is the *kung-sun,* four to five finger-widths below the ankle bone, on the inside of the foot, where the skin changes colour from pink to white. Massage it towards the anklebone. The 'warning-point' for the small intestine is the *kuan-yüan,* one hand-width (on fat people, one and a half hand-widths) above the pubic bone, over the bladder, and this should be massaged upwards. The *ho-ku* point relates to the large intestine and this lies on the back of the hand, two finger-widths below the knuckle of the forefinger, and half a finger-width towards the thumb. Massage it towards the elbow.

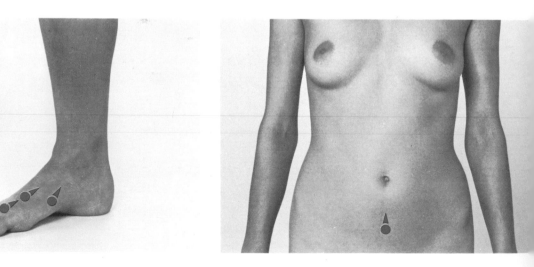

Ear acupressure

The points for the intestinal nervous system are found at the top of the hollow on the back of the ear, while those for relieving associated pains are on the outside, on the upper hollow, near the ridge. In cases of diarrhoea, the points behind and on the outside of the ear should be massaged downwards; this applies to *both* ears.

Treatment

Ear and body acupressure should be alternated daily, three to five times a day, for five to ten minutes at a time, depending on the severity of the complaint. If a virus infection is the cause, the prescribed medicines should be taken, and acupressure applied as an additional measure to relieve stomach pains.

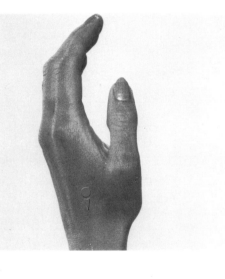

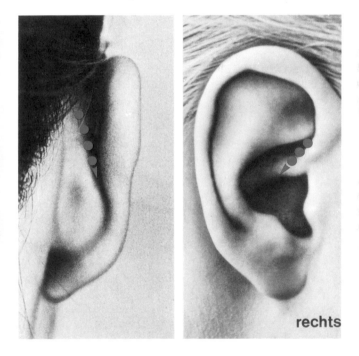

rechts

55

EMERGENCY ACUPRESSURE

Asthma attacks

If a member of your family suffers from asthma, you will probably have seen him sitting at the window, with beads of perspiration on his face, waiting for the doctor to come and give him an injection. Acupressure not only makes the wait more bearable, but can also reduce the frequency of attacks if it is regularly applied. It may be advisable to combine it with acupuncture treatment.

What are the symptoms?

An asthma attack means sudden difficulty in breathing, due to muscular spasms around the branches of the bronchial tubes in the lungs. The linings of the tubes swell up and produce phlegm.

What are the causes?

There are two main causes which, in the worst cases, can occur together. The first is chronic bronchitis which, in the asthmatic form, leads to attacks of asthma and difficulty in breathing.

Quite often, some kind of allergy is also involved, and this is the basis of the form known as allergy asthma. In these cases, any substance to which the sufferer reacts (dust, feathers, animal fur) can bring on an attack. The other form is called nervous asthma, in which an unbalanced nervous response to excitement or agitation can bring on an attack.

Body acupressure

The main point is the *shu-fu,* on the lower edge of the collarbone near the breastbone, and this should be massaged upwards. Two other points are the *chin-wei,* at the base of the breastbone, and the *tan-chung,* which lies halfway up the breastbone, level with the male nipples. Massage both upwards.

The main point of treatment for all forms of congestion in the chest is the *lieh-ch'üeh,* about two finger-widths above the base of the palm; massage it towards the base of the thumb. Relief of psychological tension occurs through the *tsu-san-li,* on the lower leg. This lies beneath the tip

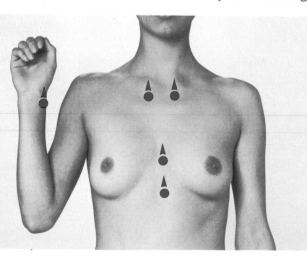

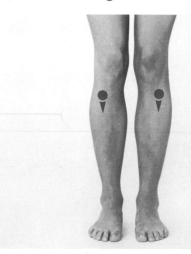

of the ring finger when the palm of the hand is placed on the kneecap, and should be massaged downwards. In cases of chronic asthma, you should also treat the *tai-chui* point, just below the prominent seventh cervical vertebra. Massage it upwards.

Ear acupressure

On the right ear, the 'point of the lungs', situated low down in the central hollow, should be massaged upwards. Another point, in the centre of the ridge surrounding the central hollow, should be massaged downwards, and the 'allergy point', just in front of the highest point of the ear, should be massaged towards the back of the head. The point for relieving psychological tension is at the upper front edge, where the ear joins the head; massage it upwards. Reverse the directions on the left ear.

What to do in an emergency

If you are on your own, as soon as you feel able to do so stand in front of a mirror and massage the ear points. If you are nervous about doing this, massage the points on the chest and arm as vigorously as possible.

If someone else is present, get them to hold the illustration against your ear to locate the points, and then to take over the massage on your ears. They can also massage the appropriate body points if you wish.

Further treatment

Ear and body acupressure should be alternated daily, one to three times a day, for five to ten minutes at a time. Do not stop taking your drugs or medicine without consulting your doctor first.

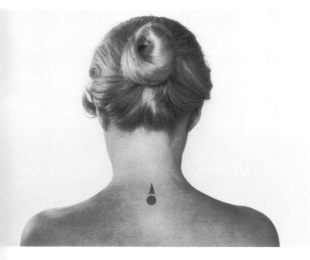

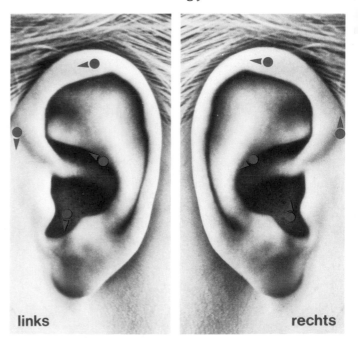

links   rechts

EMERGENCY ACUPRESSURE

Appendicitis

Of course, operation is necessary as soon as possible in a case of appendicitis, but if there is some delay acupressure will help to tide the patient over.

What are the symptoms?

Usually there are sharp pains in the right side of the stomach, low down, or in the middle of the stomach. In the early stages there is often nausea and vomiting and the tongue becomes furred. A high temperature is not necessarily a sure sign, however. A more reliable symptom is the patient's sensitivity to pressure in the general area of the appendix, one hand-width below the navel and the same distance to the right. If you press slowly down on this area, and then release the pressure quickly, the patient feels a vibrating pain. The skin over the area may also become stretched, which is a form of defence mechanism.

What is the cause?

Appendicitis results from an infection of the intestine, caused by a blockage in the appendix. If the appendix becomes sufficiently inflamed, there is a danger that it will rupture and release its contents into the abdominal cavity, giving rise to peritonitis, which is dangerous and may even be fatal. In an emergency, the inflammation should be contained as much as possible and the patient should not undertake any physical exertion whatsoever.

Body acupressure

The main point is the *lan-vee*, the so-called appendix point, six and a half finger-widths below, and two finger-widths to the outside of, the centre of the kneecap, which should be massaged downwards. Apply stronger pressure on the right leg than on the left. One and a half finger-widths lower down lies the *chü-shü*

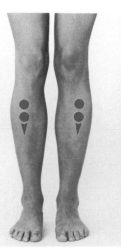
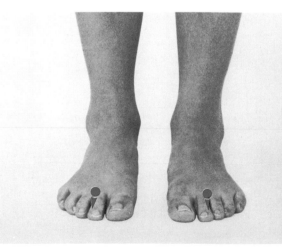

shang-lien point ('surfeit of the upper region'), which should also be massaged downwards.

The point *nei-t'ing* has a beneficial effect in containing inflammation and relieving pain. This lies just above the crease between the second and third toes, slightly nearer the second, and should be massaged towards the toes.

Finally, massage the *t'ien'shu* points, three finger-widths to each side of the navel, in a downward direction.

Ear acupressure

On the right ear, the point for the appendix is easy to find, in the middle of the valley, just above the ridge where it emerges from the central hollow. The other point, the main nerve point for the stomach, is nearby, on the ridge itself. Massage both in a forward and upward direction. On the left ear, just massage the latter point, but in the opposite direction.

What to do in an emergency

If you are alone, stand in front of a mirror and massage the ear points, as shown. If you are nervous about doing this, massage the body points, giving extra pressure to those just below the knees.

If someone else can take over, get him to hold the illustration against your ear to locate the points, and apply acupressure in the directions described. The other person can also apply body acupressure if required.

If the emergency lasts for a few days – for example, if admission to hospital is not immediately possible – apply ear and body acupressure on alternate days, massaging every two hours for five minutes at a time.

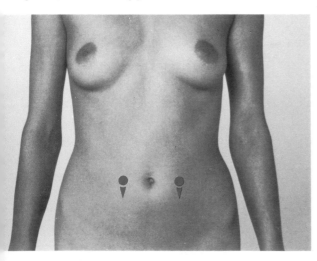

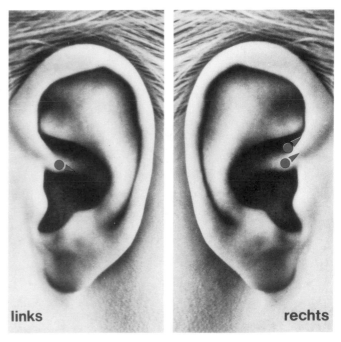

links   rechts

59

Gall bladder colic

This usually takes the form of painful cramps in the bile ducts. While it lasts, the pain is often quite severe, and afterwards there is a feeling of soreness under the right ribs.

What are the symptoms?

It is brought on by eating too much fatty food, or by agitation or irritation, making you feel uneasy, and causing you to bring up wind and even be sick. After that, the colic persists for about half an hour.

What are the causes?

The commonest cause is gallstones, which get jammed together and irritate the lining of the bile ducts. These ducts react by trying to force the stones out, and this causes the colic. It may also be due to psychological causes. One person in three suffers from gallstones, but the condition often stays 'quiet' for years, and then something happens to trigger off an attack of colic.

Body acupressure

The main point is the *dang-nang-dian,* three finger-widths below the prominent head of the outer, lower legbone (fibula). Massage it firmly in a downward direction. The other body points are complementary to this one, the first being the *tai-ch'ung,* two to three finger-widths above the crease between the big and second toes, slightly towards the former. Massage it upwards, towards the ankle.

The *yang-pai* point is on the forehead, one and a half finger-widths above each eyebrow, in line with the pupils when you are looking straight ahead. Massage it firmly upwards. The *chung-kuan* points midway between the base of the breastbone and the navel, and *shang-kuan,* two finger-widths higher up, should both be massaged upwards.

Ear acupressure

As the gall bladder and bile ducts lie on the right side of the body, you need only massage the right ear. The point for relieving pain in the bile

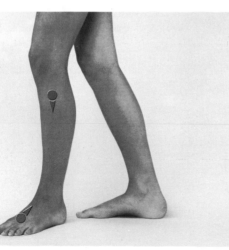

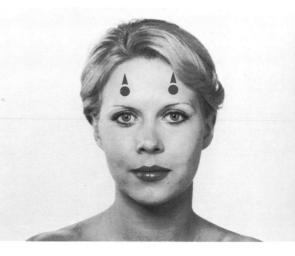

ducts lies in the upper valley of the central hollow, and should be massaged strongly forwards and upwards. The point on the back of the ear, which has the effect of reducing the muscle contractions in the lining of the gall bladder, should be massaged downwards.

What to do in an emergency

If you are on your own, massage the 'pain point of the bile ducts' on the ear, as strongly as possible; this is particularly effective. If you have no mirror, and cannot locate the point, massage firmly the point on each side of the forehead. Sometimes the pain will prevent you from bending over and reaching the point on the lower leg, but if you can, this is also very effective.

If someone else can apply the acupressure, he should place the book next to your ear, to locate the points, and massage them vigorously. If he also takes over the body acupressure, he should massage the point on the lower leg especially strongly.

Further treatment

If you are inclined to have gall bladder colic, you should see your doctor about having an operation on the gall bladder. Apart from acupressure, a hot, wet compress applied to the area gives relief. If you want to avoid gallstones altogether you should ensure that you have a properly balanced diet.

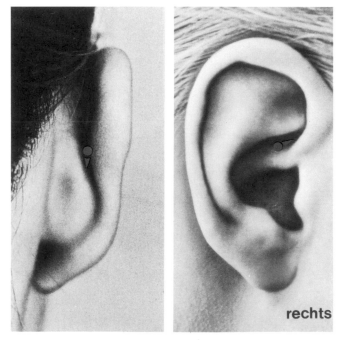

rechts

61

EMERGENCY ACUPRESSURE

Heart pains

Throughout the Western world, heart pains are symptomatic of the most serious of all common illnesses. They may signify an attack of angina pectoris (a weakness of the heart muscle) or, if severe, coronary thrombosis (heart attack). There may be several minor heart attacks before a major one occurs.

If you suspect any of these, you must see your doctor immediately, so that he can carry out an electrocardiogram (E.C.G.) and other tests to diagnose the exact cause. If the condition seems serious he will admit you to hospital and may even put you under intensive care.

What are the symptoms?

Heart pains range from a slight stab in the left side of the chest to really severe pains.

What are the causes?

Heart pains always stem from a lack of oxygen in the heart; psychological tension or agitation have the effect of making the pain worse. There are essentially two different forms: angina pectoris and coronary thrombosis, in which the lack of oxygen in the affected part of the heart last so long that it dies. Other parts of the body, given a period of rest, are able to regenerate themselves after an illness, but for the heart there can be no rest at all. The greater the dead area of the heart, the more dangerous it is for the patient.

Body acupressure

The first point is the *tung-li* ('link with the inner self') which lies on the inner arm, two finger-widths above the base of the palm in line with the little finger. Massage it towards the little finger. Next, the *shao-chong* point, which stimulates the heart and which lies on the inside of the little finger near the base of the nail, should be massaged across the finger, from the inside out, just below the nail.

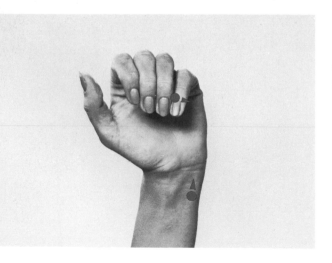

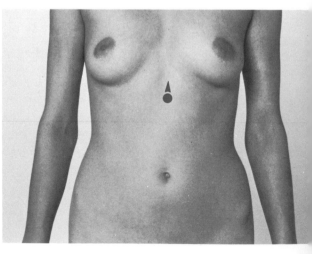

The *chü-ch'üeh,* the 'alarm point for the heart', which is two (if you are fat, three to four) finger-widths below the base of the breastbone, should be massaged upwards. In combination with this point, you should also massage the *hsin-shu,* the 'point of equilibrium of the heart'. This is on the back, two to three finger-widths to each side of the fifth dorsal vertebra, and should be massaged downwards.

Ear acupressure

As the heart is on the left side, you need only massage the left ear. The 'pain point' of the heart is on the flat part of the ear, just above the central hollow; massage it downwards. The 'strengthening point' of the heart is in the hollow behind the ear and should be massaged upwards.

What to do in an emergency

If you are on your own, use a mirror to locate the first of the ear points, which is particularly effective, and massage it strongly. If there is no mirror handy, massage the points on the arm and chest as vigorously as possible. If someone else is present, get him to hold the illustration against your ear to locate the points, and massage strongly, as shown.

If, for some reason, you cannot be admitted to hospital for some days, you should apply ear and body acupressure on alternate days, every two hours, for five to ten minutes at a time.

Further treatment

Acupressure is beneficial until the doctor is able to take over.

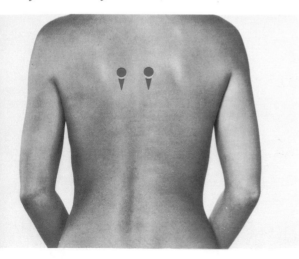

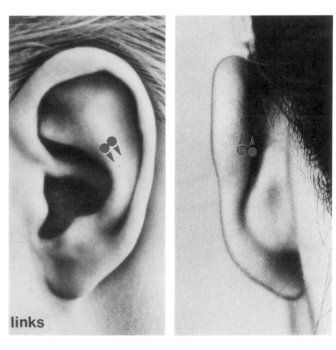

links

EMERGENCY ACUPRESSURE

Kidney pains

Acupressure helps to relieve kidney pain and eases the period of waiting until medical attention can be given.

What are the symptoms?

Kidney pain is due to a stone which, if it is still in the kidney, has its worst effects in the back, around the hips. If the stone is in the ureter, between the kidneys and the bladder, the spread of pain is deeper, more to the side and in the bladder itself.

What are the causes?

The most usual cause of pain is a kidney stone, it can also be due to fragments of inflamed lining which have broken away, though this is much less common. There are various kinds of kidney stone, some of which can be dissolved, given the right conditions. If you have kidney pains you should obviously see your doctor immediately.

Body acupressure

The *ching-men* point, which is the 'alarm point' of the kidneys, is at the open end of the twelfth rib. You will find it by placing your bent arm against your body and measuring four finger-widths back from the point of the elbow.

There is another point nearby which is useful for pains in the side: called the *tai-mo*, it is located three finger-widths below, and three finger-widths forward from the previous point. Massage both in a forward and downward direction.

If the pain is deeper and to the side, massage the *wu-shu* point, near the prominent part of the ilium, or hip bone, in a downward direction.

In combination with these, especially the first, the *ching-men*, you should massage the *shen-shu* point, the 'stimulus point' of the kidneys. This lies two to two and a half finger-widths to each side of the base of the second lumbar vertebra, and should be massaged downwards.

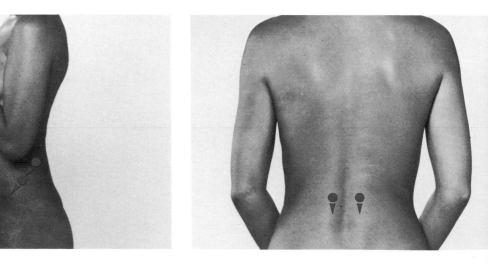

The general point for easing cramps is the *t-ai-ch'ung*, two to three finger-widths above the crease between the big toe and the second toe, slightly towards the former. Massage it upwards.

Ear acupressure

On the right ear, massage all the way up the inside front fold, from the 'bladder point' to the 'kidney point'. If you have pains in the left side, massage the same points on the left ear but from top to bottom (not illustrated). These are the 'pain points' of the ureter, between the kidneys and the bladder, and of the kidneys themselves.

To reduce the muscular cramps which occur with kidney pains, massage the appropriate point behind each ear, situated at the top where it joins the head. Massage it downwards on the right ear, upwards on the left.

What to do in an emergency

If you are on your own, it is especially effective to massage the ear points as strongly as possible. If you have no mirror handy and cannot locate the ear points, massage the points on the side of the body instead and, if you can reach them, those on the feet as well, again using firm pressure.

Someone else could hold the illustration of the ear next to your own right ear, locate the points, and massage them vigorously. If necessary, the equivalent points on the left ear should be massaged in the opposite directions. The body points can also be massaged if you wish.

As a general rule, include plenty of liquid in your diet, and make sure that the air is reasonably moist, both at home and at work.

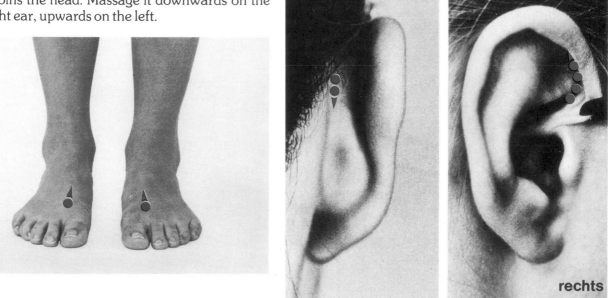

rechts

65

EMERGENCY ACUPRESSURE

Toothache

Toothache is very common and often seems to occur when you cannot get to a dentist, which means putting up with it until you can be treated. Acupressure is beneficial here, and can also be used after a visit to a dentist which has involved a lot of drilling, leaving the nerve of the tooth on edge. Of course, you can take pain-relieving tablets for toothache but you may not have them handy. Some people find these too strong for them, anyway.

What are the symptoms?

The pains are usually localized in one tooth at first, then spread throughout the whole of that part of the jaw. In severe cases, both upper and lower jaws can be affected. If the pain throbs excessively you should go to a dentist or dental clinic as soon as is practical.

What are the causes?

Toothache is a sign of an irritated nerve. There are a number of causes, such as an infected tooth or a filling. You need proper dental treatment in such cases, and should not regard acupressure as a substitute for it, or as an excuse to postpone it, even though you may not like going to the dentist. You can use acupressure during a course of dental treatment to relieve the pain.

Body acupressure

The main point is the *shang-yang,* near the lower outside corner of the index fingernail (on the side nearest the thumb). Massage it towards the knuckle. The supplementary points are the *hsia-kuan,* in a little hollow on the cheekbone just above the hinge of the jawbone, and the *chia-ch'e,* on the point of the jaw. Massage both upwards.

The *ti-ts'ang* point, one finger-width from the edge of the mouth, should be massaged downwards. The *ch'üan-chiao* point is particularly effective for pains in the upper jaw. It is situated in a small hollow, just below the point of the

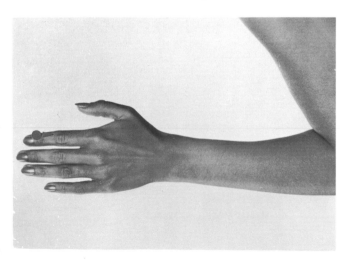

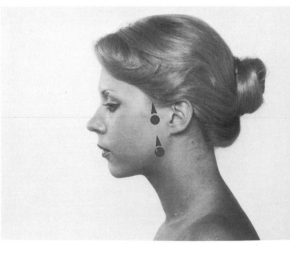

cheekbone, in line with the outside corner of the eye. Massage it towards the ear.

Ear acupressure

The 'tooth point' is on the lobe, towards the back, midway between the edge of the ear and the central hollow. On the right ear it should be massaged upwards and backwards, on the left ear forwards and downwards. Massage the ear on the side where the pain is; if you are uncertain about this, massage both ears.

What to do in an emergency

The ear points are especially effective in combating toothache, so massage these as strongly as possible. If, for some reason, you cannot do this, the most important point to massage is the one on the forefinger. Keep on with this throughout your course of dental treatment, always using plenty of pressure.

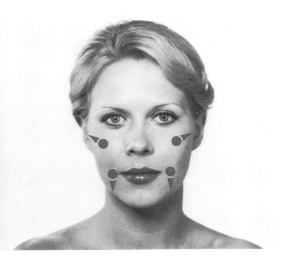

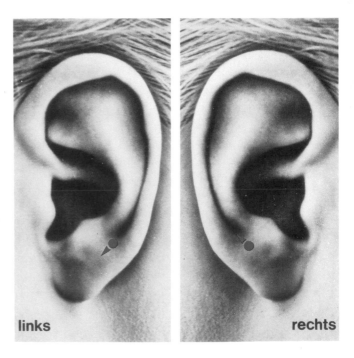

links   rechts

67

EMERGENCY ACUPRESSURE

Flatulence

A certain amount of gas forms naturally during the digestive process, but this does not cause discomfort since it is usually absorbed through the intestinal wall.

What are the symptoms?

First, there is a 'rumbling' sensation in the intestines, then the gas finds it way to its natural outlet.

What are the causes?

Flatulence is gas which is caused either by swallowing too much air, or which forms in excess during the digestive process. It is normal, when eating, for a small amount of air to be swallowed, but nervous or depressed individuals tend to take in more. So if you tend towards flatulence try the acupressure appropriate to this condition and alternate it with the appropriate treatment for depression or nervousness (see pages 52 or 114).

Flatulence can also be caused by the pancreas or the gall bladder, in which case the appropriate treatment will be found on pages 120 and 73 respectively. Certain heart diseases may also lead to flatulence. A medical examination should decide which of the possible causes applies in your particular case: then practise acupressure in consultation with your doctor.

Body acupressure

First, there is the Chinese point *ho-ku* which strengthens the activity of the large intestine (in this case, gas absorption): it lies two finger-widths below the knuckle joint of the index-finger, and half a finger-width towards the thumb, and should be massaged towards the elbow. You should also treat the next Chinese point for the colon, the *san-li,* about three finger-widths below the crease of the elbow, when the arm is bent: massage the arm upwards.

Stimulation of the small intestine is achieved by massaging the *hou-hsi* point on the edge of the palm below the knuckle joint of the little finger: massage it towards the arm. You should also treat the *nei-kuan* point, three finger-widths above the base of the palm and in the centre of the lower arm: apply acupressure towards the palm of the hand.

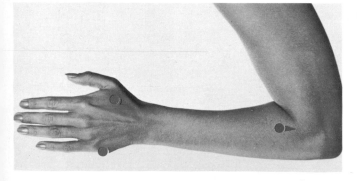
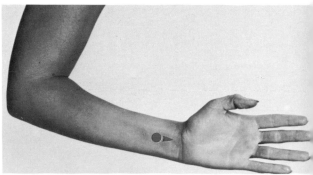

Finally there is the point known as 'over-abundance of the upper region' (Chinese name, *chü-shü shang-lien)* which is eight finger-widths below the centre of the kneecap, and two finger-widths towards the outside of the leg. Massage it downwards.

Ear acupressure

On the right ear you should treat the solar plexus, the nerve centre of the abdomen, which is situated on the ridge at the point where it emerges from the central hollow: massage it upwards and forwards. Immediately above it, near the underside of the ridge, lie the points for the pancreas, the gall bladder, and the small and large intestines, which should also be massaged upwards and forwards. Finally, there is the point of psychological relief, at the forward, upper edge of ear: massage it upwards. On the left ear the directions of massage should be reversed, as shown.

Treatment

Ear acupressure and body acupressure should be alternated daily, one to three times a day, for ten to fifteen minutes depending on the severity of the complaint. If it is necessary to massage the appropriate points for nervousness or depression, or stimulate the gall bladder or pancreas, this should be done at different times. Avoid foods which cause a build-up of gas, such as pulses (beans, peas, lentils), onions, and cabbage.

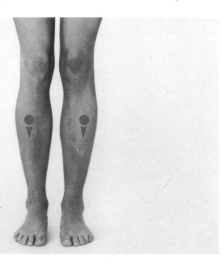

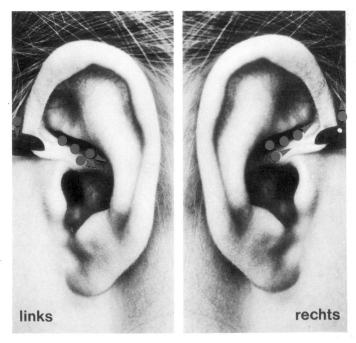

links   rechts

Forgetfulness and lack of concentration

These complaints are found at all levels; school-children, workers under stress, the elderly find it hard to concentrate at times. Their ability to remember things may also leave a lot to be desired.

What are the symptoms?

Schoolchildren find it hard to retain what they have learnt, or are so inattentive and fidgety that they are unable to concentrate in class or learn their lessons. Forgetfulness in older people begins when they find, to their surprise, that quite recent events have gone out of their minds, whereas earlier incidents are still clearly remembered.

A lack of concentration shows when some-one fails to do something he has said he would do, although motivation may play a part here, depending on whether he does a thing freely or against his will.

What are the causes?

Often, young people have never learnt to concentrate all their attention on something and quickly forget what they have just heard. On the other hand, in serious cases, there may be a failure in the functioning of the brain, which requires examination and diagnosis by a specialist. In the elderly, forgetfulness and the loss of concentration can be put down to the brain getting tired, and in this case the doctor will usually prescribe stimulating drugs. Combined with these, acupressure is very beneficial.

Body acupressure

The main points on the body are the *pai-hui,* in the centre of the skull, on an imaginary line between the ears, and four surrounding points ('wisdom of the four gods'), one and a half to two finger-widths distant, forwards, backwards, and on each side. Massage all these points

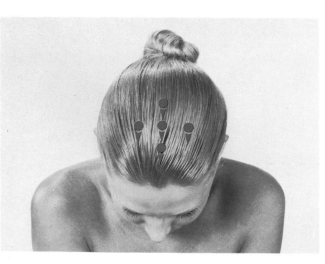

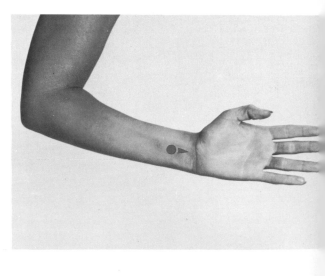

towards the forehead. Next, there is the *nei-kuan* ('inner barrier') point, in the centre of the lower, inner arm, three finger-widths above the base of the palm. Massage it towards the hand. Finally, massage the main energy point, the *ch'i-hai* ('sea of energy'), two to three (on fat people, four to five) finger-widths below the navel. The direction, in this case, is upwards.

Ear acupressure

On the ear, the first point for concentration is situated above and slightly to the rear of the centre of the lobe. Massage it upwards and backwards. Next, there is the central point for nervous energy, which lies on the ridge, where it emerges from the central hollow; massage it upwards and forwards. Finally, massage the front of the ear, where it joins the head, from bottom to top. All these directions apply to the right ear. Reverse them on the left ear.

Treatment

Ear and body acupressure should be alternated daily, once to three times a day, for five to ten minutes, depending on the seriousness of the problem. If you are taking drugs or medicine, you should only reduce or stop taking them in consultation with your doctor.

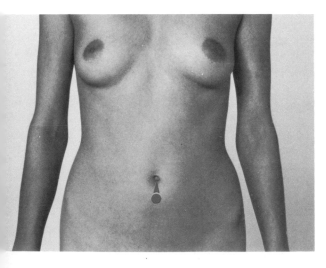

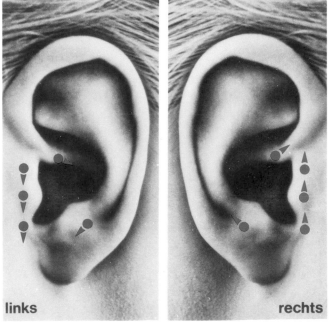

links   rechts

71

Gall bladder malfunction

Many people suffer from gallstones and complain about stomach pains or a dull ache under the ribs on the right-hand side, especially after eating fatty foods. Most gall bladder complaints start with a functional weakness of some sort and, in such cases, acupressure can help to stimulate the functions and prevent more serious problems.

What are the symptoms?

The main purpose of bile salts is to emulsify fats in the small intestine – that is, to break down into such minute drops that they can be absorbed by the intestine's mucous membrane. If bile is lacking, the normal brown colour of the stools fades, almost to the colour of concrete, and this is a sign of a serious illness. If you have this symptom, go to your doctor straight-away.

In less obvious cases, the most probable cause is distortion of the bile duct, which produces a dull ache in the region of the gall bladder, spreading downwards towards the back. Another frequent symptom is headaches (see the section on page 100).

What is the cause?

One of the main causes is a person's mental state (traditionally the gall bladder was known as 'the seat of the temperament'). Malfunction may also be due to inflammation or a gallstone. In any case, see your doctor and get a proper diagnosis. He will probably prescribe certain drugs and put you on a diet; you should combine this treatment with acupressure in consultation with him.

Body acupressure

The key point for the gall bladder is the *dang-nang-dian,* three finger-widths below the top of the outer legbone (fibula). Next, there is the *kuang-ming* point, about one and a half hand-widths above the outer tip of the anklebone. Apply firm massage to both points in a downward direction.

Two other points, which have a more direct effect, are the *chung-kuan* and the *shang-kuan,* the first half way between the navel and the

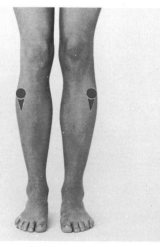
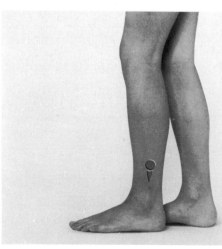

bottom of the breastbone, and the second two finger-widths above. Both should be massaged upwards.

Ear acupressure

The gall bladder point on the right ear is just above the place where the ridge emerges from the central hollow. This should be massaged strongly upwards and forwards. The same applies to the central nerve point, which is in the middle of the ridge where it emerges from the central hollow. There is a further point, at the top and to the front of the ear lobe, which should be massaged upwards.

On the left ear, the central nerve point should be massaged downwards and backwards and, if required, the 'point of care', which is at the centre front of the lobe, should be massaged downwards. The 'point of care' is often over-looked as the reason for a number of complaints, especially stomach cramp and heartburn. Finally, the point at the top-front of the ear lobe should be massaged downwards.

Treatment

Carry out ear and body acupressure on alternate days, one to three times a day, for five to ten minutes, depending on the severity of the complaint. As a preventative measure, treatment every two or three days should be enough. Follow your doctor's instructions regarding dieting and the medicines he has prescribed, and consult him about gradually reducing the amount you need to take.

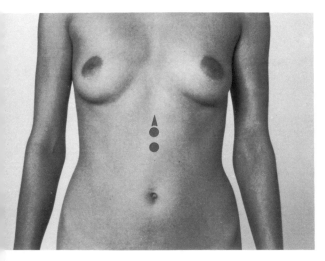

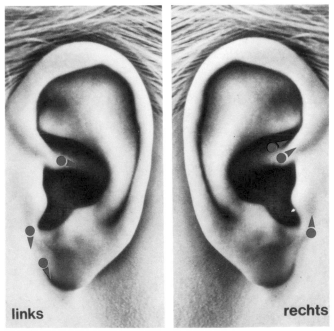

links   rechts

73

Haemorrhoids (piles)

This is a common complaint, particularly among people with a sedentary occupation. It should be said that our practice of using toilet paper must be partly responsible because in countries where tradition calls for the use of water alone, haemorrhoids are almost unknown.

What are the symptoms?

They usually start with the patient having an irresistible itching in the anus. Subsequently, in the case of external piles, he will notice that there is a small swelling in the anus, near the sphincter. Internal haemorrhoids, on the other hand, can only be reached by a rectal examination by a doctor. In some cases of haemorrhoids there is no pain, while in others they bleed from time to time, especially when the motions are hard.

What is the cause?

The usual cause is a weakness in the tissue which connects the blood vessels, as in the case with varicose veins. The blood vessels which, by

swelling up, serve the purpose of supporting the sphincter and forming a gas-tight closure, get out of condition, become distended and appear in the form of piles.

Body acupressure

The first point is the *chang-men,* which will be found by placing the bent arm against the body and locating the point directly beneath the elbow, on the side of the body. Massage it forwards and upwards. There are two other points: the *ch'ü-ch'üan,* on the inside of the fold of the knee, which should be massaged upwards, and the *wei-chung,* level with it, and in the centre of the fold of the knee, which should be massaged downwards. Lastly, there is a point on the skull, the *pai-hui,* lying in the centre of an imaginary line between the ears; massage it towards the front.

Ear-acupressure

Treatment of the ears is particularly effective. The haemorrhoid point is hidden in the ear, inside the fold of the rising ridge, where it turns

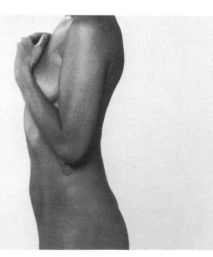 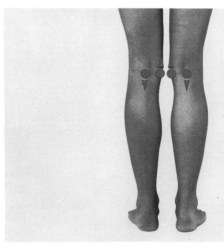

towards the circular ridge surrounding the central hollow. Firmly massage the point upwards on the right ear, and downwards on the left ear.

Treatment

Ear acupressure, in this instance, is more effec-tive than body acupressure, so apply the former two or three days running, once or twice a day, for five minutes, then body acupressure for one day. If you can find a doctor who specializes in treatment of haemorrhoids (a proctologist), you should discuss acupressure with him. Also, after passing a motion, first use a ball of cottonwool soaked in lukewarm water, dry the area, then rub in a suitable ointment. Do this in addition to acupressure.

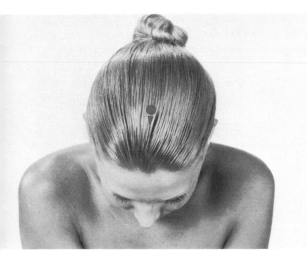

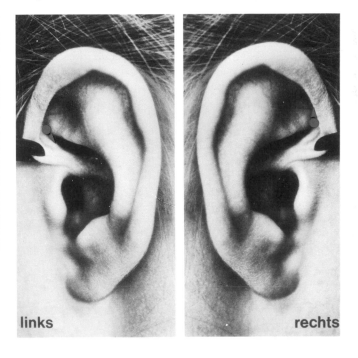

links   rechts

Hay fever

Hay fever usually develops in childhood and is found mainly among people living in towns and cities. It starts in late spring and, if severe, often lasts right through the summer. Bad cases of hay fever can eventually lead to bronchitis and even asthma.

What are its symptoms?

Hay fever is a basically a heavy, allergy-based cold, with a runny nose, sore eyes, and compulsive sneezing.

What is its cause?

It is caused by an allergy to pollen, which is why the hay fever season coincides with the period when plants are in bloom. It is possible that a certain gland, the thymus, acts as an irritant and is partly to blame for the allergic reaction. In severe cases, doctors prescribe cortisone sprays and tablets. Acupressure can be applied, in consultation with your doctor, as a means of reducing the need for tablets.

Body acupressure

First, the *ho-ku* point, on the back of the hand, two finger-widths below the knuckle of the forefinger, and half a finger-width towards the thumb, should be massaged towards the elbow. Next there are the points *ying-hsiang* ('receiver of scents and smells'), situated close to the middle of each side of the nose, at the top end of the line between the nose and the corner of the mouth, and *ho-chiao,* one and a half finger-widths lower down. Massage both in an upward direction.

The *inn-trang* point, in the centre of the bridge of the nose, between the eyebrows, should be massaged downwards. Finally, there are two more points, lying close together, both of which should be massaged upwards. These are the *ching-ming,* on each side of the bridge, at the point which supports a pair of glasses, and *ts'uan-chu,* at the inner end of each eyebrow.

Ear acupressure

On the right ear, the 'allergy-point', at the highest point of the ear, should be massaged

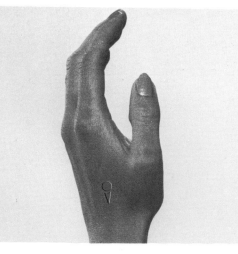
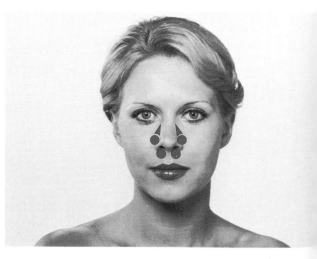

from front to back. There is also a point in the wall of the turn of the ear ('thymus point'), which should be massaged downwards. Finally, there is the 'nose point', situated at the base, and to the front, of the ear lobe. This should be massaged forwards and upwards. The same points are used on the left ear, but massage should be applied in the opposite direction in each case.

Treatment

Ear and body acupressure should be alternated daily, one to three times a day, for periods of five to ten minutes, depending on the severity of the case. If acupressure proves ineffective at the beginning of the pollen season, it is a good idea to visit an acupuncturist. He will apply needles to the appropriate points, and the subsequent improvement can be maintained by self-applied acupressure. This, in turn, will bring about further improvement and may, if your doctor agrees, eventually lead to a gradual withdrawal of cortisone treatment.

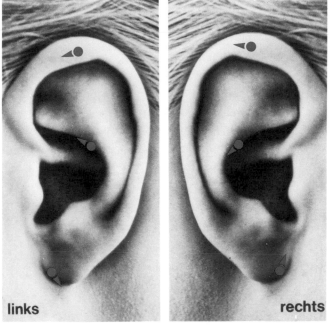

links   rechts

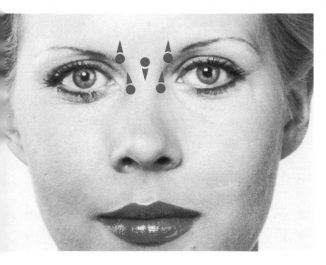

Hearing defects

As you get older, the functions of the ear tend to deteriorate, giving rise to hardness of hearing or buzzing in the ears. Acupressure cannot cure these complaints but it can lessen the problem, or help to delay or prevent any worsening of your condition.

What are the symptoms?

You become aware of the problem when you have to keep asking people to repeat what they have just said. An E.N.T. (ear, nose and throat) specialist can measure your hearing ability with an audiogram. Sometimes elderly people get a persistent buzzing or ringing in the ears which causes considerable discomfort and is, unfortunately, incurable as a rule.

What are the causes?

The ears need a constant supply of blood but as you get older the circulation tends to weaken. An examination by an E.N.T. specialist will determine the exact cause of your ear trouble, and your acupressure treatment should be carried out in consultation with him. It is quite likely that your hearing will improve if the loss of circulation is not too great.

Body acupressure

The key point of the ear is the *eh-men* ('the door of the ear'), which lies in front of the ear, in a hollow which forms when you open your mouth slightly. Massage it forwards and upwards.

In conjunction with this, the Chinese massage the *wai-kuan* point, midway between the tip of the middle finger and the point of elbow. Massage it strongly towards the elbow. There is an equivalent point on the inner arm, the *nei-kuan* ('inner barrier'), which lies three finger-widths above the base of the palm, on the centre line of the arm. Massage it towards the fingers.

For low blood pressure you should also massage the *chung-ch'ung* point, just below the lower corner of the middle fingernail nearest the index finger. Massage the finger below the nail, from the index finger side towards the ring finger. If you have high blood pressure, use only light pressure.

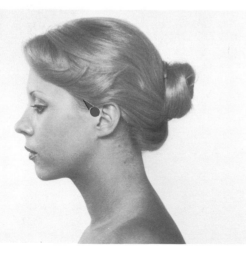

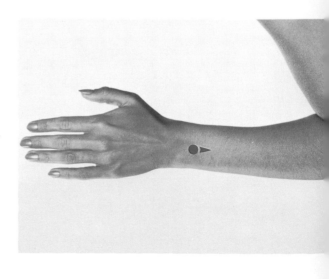

Ear acupressure

The main point on the ear is situated in the middle of the vertical ridge, in front of the central hollow. It stimulates the function of the auditory nerve, and should be massaged upwards on the right ear. There is another point, fairly high up and towards the back of the lobe, which should be massaged in an upward and backward direction. On the left ear, the points are the same, but massage should be applied in the opposite direction in each case.

Treatment

Ear and body acupressure should be alternated daily. Any drugs or medicines prescribed by your doctor should be taken as well.

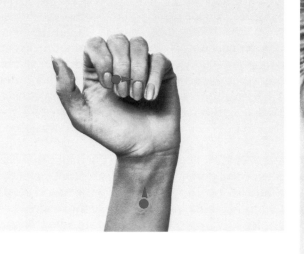

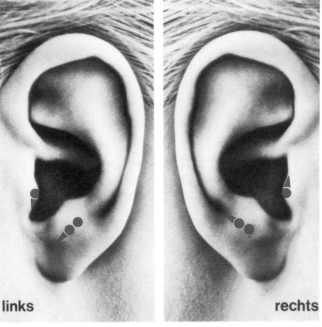

links   rechts

79

Heart palpitations

The nervous heart

You are not normally aware of your heartbeat, but if you get excited or agitated, or indulge in physical exertion, you feel it beating strongly. If this sensation occurs frequently or persistently, something is wrong.

What are the symptoms?

There is a feeling of unease or anxiety around the heart, which may be quite pronounced, together with an uneven heartbeat and an uncomfortable pressure in the area, especially after a period of excitement. Other symptoms which may accompany marked palpitations are giddiness, a fast pulse, sweating, loss of balance, and broken sleep.

What are the causes?

Palpitations result from a combination of nervousness and excitement in a person of a certain disposition. There are other causes, such as the after-effects of influenza, or a serious illness or operation. What is essentially affected is the heart's nervous system, and an accurate diagnosis by a doctor is necessary to establish that the patient is not suffering from a serious heart condition or an over-active thyroid gland. Practise acupressure in consultation with your doctor.

Body acupressure

The first point is the *tung-li* (meaning 'union with the interior'), on the inside of the lower arm, two finger-widths above the base of the palm, on an imaginary line extended from the little finger. Massage towards the latter. Next, two points – the *chiu-wei*, at the base of the breastbone, and the *ta-chung,* in the centre of the breastbone, level with a man's nipples (two finger-widths below the halfway point of the breastbone) – should both be massaged upwards.

For psychological relief, massage the *tsu-san-li* point downwards. This is found by placing the hand on the kneecap, so that the middle finger is touching the skin: the point lies immediately beneath the tip of the ring finger, on the lower leg.

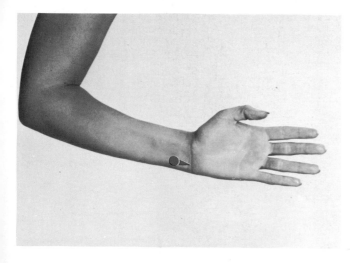

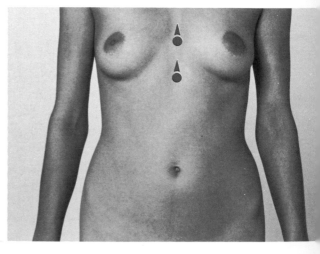

Ear acupressure

As the heart is on the left side of the body, only the left ear is treated. The main point for the nerves of the heart is on the lower edge of the central hollow, where the ridge starts. Massage it upwards. A second point, in the middle of the fleshy part of the upper ear, helps relaxation and should be massaged towards the back of the head. The motor point for the heart lies in the hollow behind the ear and should be massaged upwards.

Treatment

Ear and body acupressure should be alternated daily; as a rule, one or two treatments a day lasting five to ten minutes are sufficient. If you are taking any drugs or medicines for the heart, you must not reduce them without consulting your doctor.

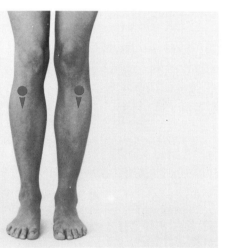

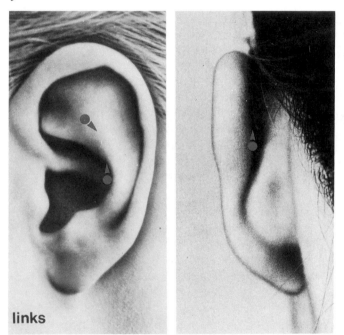

links

Heart weakness

Many old people suffer from a weak heart and need the support of drugs or medicines. They should continue to take these, but if they also use acupressure to strengthen the heart, they will feel noticeably stronger.

What are the symptoms of a weak heart?

With the slightest exertion, such as climbing stairs, the patient gets breathless, his lips turn blue, and he has to stop and take a breather before going on. An early indication is a need to get up in the night to urinate, which was not there before. This is because at night, when the heart is not so loaded, the kidneys receive more blood and are able to produce urine.

The doctor can measure the extent to which the heart is weakened by taking an electro-cardiogram (E.C.G.), while the patient rides a bicycling machine or performs some other exercise. The electrical curves made by the heart, in relation to the loading, show the extent of the weakness.

What are the causes?

The heart has to work very hard. In the course of a day enough blood to fill a tanker is pumped from the heart and through the veins. This goes on day and night, year in, year out, and when the body is exerted, or put under stress, the heart has to beat three times as fast as when the body is at rest. No wonder it gets weaker with age! In such cases, the doctor will prescribe drugs called glycosides to strengthen the heart, and these should still be taken in addition to the acupressure treatment.

Body acupressure

The stimulus point for the heart (and psyche), the *shao-chong,* lies at the inside lower corner of the little fingernail and should be massaged below the nail, from the inside out. Next comes the *tung-li* point, on the inside of the lower arm, two finger-widths above the base of the palm, on an imaginary line extended from the little finger. Massage towards the latter. There is also

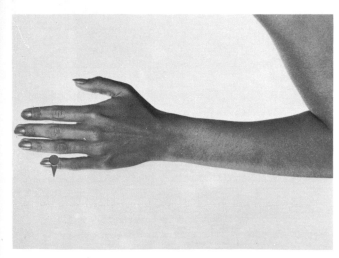

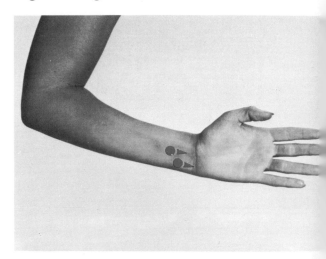

the *nei-kuan* point (meaning 'inner barrier'), in the middle of the inside lower arm, three finger-widths above the palm, which should be massaged towards the fingers. Lastly, the points *chiu-wei,* at the base of the breastbone, and *tan-chung* in the centre of the breastbone, on a level with a man's nipples, should be massaged upwards.

Ear acupressure

As the heart lies on the left side of the body, only the left ear should have treatment. The point associated with the heart muscles, which lies in the hollow behind the ear, should be firmly massaged. The point on the outside of the ear acts against contractions of the heart, and should be massaged backwards and downwards.

Treatment

Ear and body acupressure should be alternated daily, two or three times a day, depending on the condition. The usual drugs must still be taken. The advantage of acupressure here lies, not in being able to reduce the drug intake, but in increasing the patient's energy, which should be used sparingly.

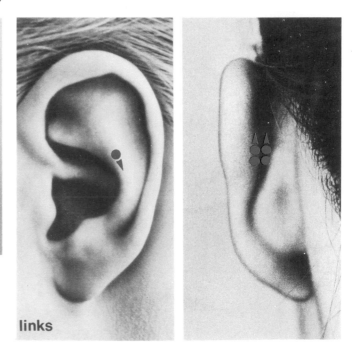

links

83

Hip pains

Hip pains are quite common, due to wear on the joint (arthrosis), or inflammation (arthritis). A badly damaged joint cannot be cured but can now be replaced with a steel joint. In less severe cases, acupressure can help to relieve the pain.

What are the symptoms?

The first sign is a feeling of stiffness and numbness. As the condition worsens, when you walk or even when sitting down, you get a pain in the side at hip level, which shoots inwards towards the groin or down the leg. If you walk for some time, or go up stairs, the pain gets noticeably worse. Such pains are often mistaken for sciatica or rheumatism. Sometimes the joint swells up, especially if you exert yourself unduly. You may also hear a grinding noise when you move. Later on, leg movement becomes restricted, particularly if both hips are

affected; spreading the legs apart is very painful indeed.

What is the cause?

The main reason is wear on the cartilage in the joint. As you grow older, this process increases, which is why old people suffer most, but it can be accelerated by obesity or strenuous sporting activity. In women, the loss of hormone secretion from the ovaries after the menopause is a contributory cause.

Unfortunately, cartilage is a substance which does not renew itself, as other parts of the body do, yet, in the large joints it bears a considerable strain and is subject to great wear and tear, which is only kept to a minimum by the lubricating fluid in the joint. However, if this fluid is of the wrong composition, or inflames the joint, there is much greater wear on the cartilage, and

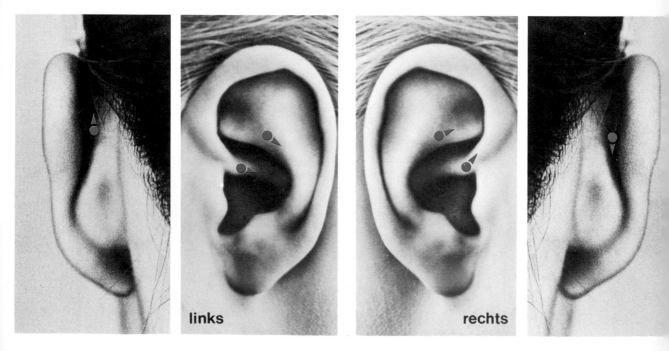

links

rechts

hip pains result. The usual treatment is injections, sometimes directly into the joint itself, and pills. This should be combined with acupressure, in consultation with your doctor.

Body acupressure

No body acupressure is recommended for this complaint; ear acupressure is much more effective.

Ear-acupressure

Even if only one joint gives pain, apply acupressure to both ears, but massage the one on the affected side more firmly. The 'pain point' for the hip joint is situated at the tip of a small, triangular hollow in the upper part of the ear, and on the right ear should be massaged forwards and upwards.

Next, the 'energy point' for the central nerve area, which is located where the ridge of the ear emerges from the central hollow, should be massaged firmly in an upward direction. In the left ear reverse the directions.

For loss of movement of the hip-joint, massage the corresponding point on the back of the ear, in the upper hollow; on the right ear downwards, and on the left ear upwards.

Treatment

Ear acupressure alone is used. You should massage with firm pressure, every day or possibly every other day. During the period of treatment, rest the joint as much as possible and do not move around too much. If you are overweight, go on a diet, and refer to the section on addictions (page 22).

Hoarseness

Hoarseness is a symptom of too much talking, singing or smoking, or may be associated with a cold. Treatment by acupressure merely brings relief.

What are the symptoms?

You are said to be suffering from hoarseness when you have a rasping, croaky voice, or you lose it altogether.

What are the causes?

Hoarseness is caused by inflamed vocal cords due to overstrain from singing or talking (especially if you are unused to it), or from smoking too much. The inflammation may also be due to an infection, such as a cold or influenza. If it lasts more than three or four days, it may signal a more serious illness, and you should visit your doctor without delay.

Body acupressure

There are two local points, which are easily found if you tilt your head slightly backwards. The first, the *jen-ying* (meaning 'friendly greeting') is one finger-width above the upper edge of the adam's apple, while the second, the *shui-t'u*, is two finger-widths below the first. Massage both downwards.

The key point for all throat complaints is the *shao-shang*, which is on the outside edge of the thumb, next to the base of the nail. Massage it across the back of the thumb, just below the nail, from the outside in.

The point which strengthens the vocal cords is the *chung-chu*, which lies on the back of the hand, one finger-width below the middle of the knuckle of the ring finger and half a finger-width towards the little finger. Massage it towards the elbow.

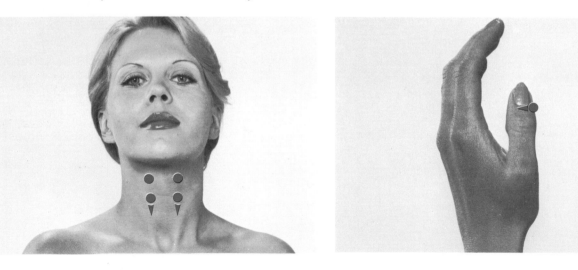

Ear acupressure

The point associated with the vocal cords is on the outside of the ear, at the back of the lobe. Massage it upwards and backwards on the right ear, downwards and forwards on the left. There is another point, similarly placed, but on the back of the ear, which is associated with the muscular fibres of the vocal cords. On the right ear this should be massaged upwards, and on the left, downwards.

Treatment

Alternate ear and body acupressure daily, one to three times a day, for five to ten minutes at a time, depending on the severity of the complaint.

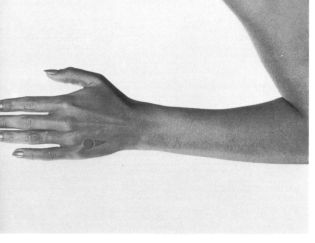

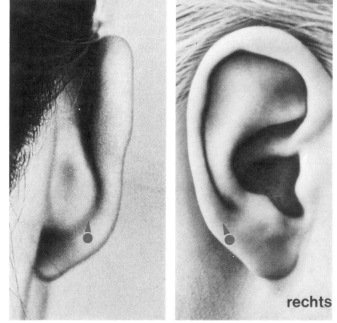

rechts

87

Hormonal troubles in women

1 Menstrual irregularities

Many women, especially when they are young, have trouble with their periods. Their hormone secretion lacks stability, giving rise to irregular periods and menstrual pains. Acupressure helps to stabilize the situation.

What are its symptoms?

Instead of the normal monthly cycle of 27 to 28 days, periods occur at irregular intervals. The hormonal weakness can also cause variations in bleeding – there may be too much or too little – and it may often be painful as well.

What is its cause?

In young women, the whole hormonal system needs 'tuning up'. The tendency is for it to stabilize itself gradually, especially after the birth of the first child. Frequently, however, this does not occur and psychological causes may play an important part. In all cases, the cause should be diagnosed by a gynecologist, and acupressure carried out in consultation with him.

Body acupressure

The *k'o-chu-jen* point is situated at the top of the jawbone, in a little hollow which is formed when the mouth is open, two finger-widths in front of the ear; it has a regulating influence on the central hormone system. Massage it upwards.

For all complaints in the region of the pelvis, the *san-yin-chiao* point should be used. This lies three to four finger-widths above the point of the inner anklebone, at the back of the shinbone, and should be massaged upwards.

Finally, there is the *ch'i-hai* point, which is a general energy point and also has a more direct, stimulating effect on the appropriate functions. This lies two or three finger-widths below the

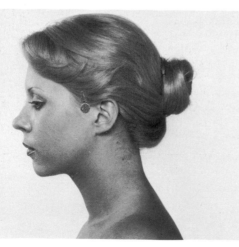

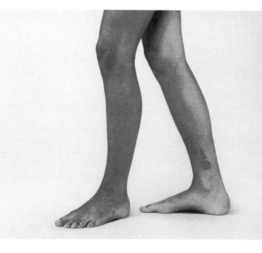

navel (on fat people, four to five), and should be massaged upwards.

Ear acupressure

On the right ear, locate the points for the ovaries and the womb, which lie in the channel within the ridge of the ear, where it emerges from the central hollow, and massage them well towards the top of the ear. On the left ear, massage the same point downwards.

Note that these points lie right inside the fold: if you compare the channel with the letter U, you will find them at the bottom and on the upper, inner wall of the U.

Treatment

Ear and body acupressure should be alternated daily, one to three times a day. Massage the points firmly a few days before the period, and more gently during the period.

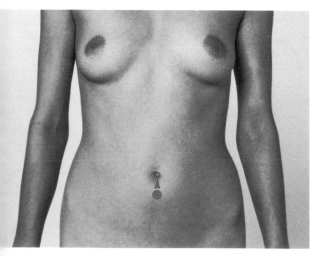

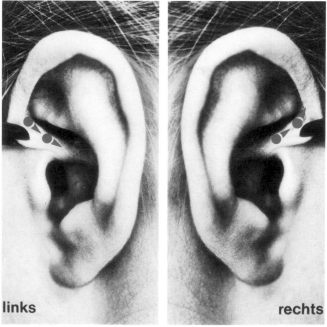

links   rechts

Hormonal troubles in women

2 Menopausal problems – hot flushes

The menopause begins at about forty-five to fifty, when monthly periods cease. A lot of women have difficulties at this time of life, until they get adjusted to the new hormonal situation, both physically and mentally. In such cases, acupressure helps to relieve the various problems.

What are the symptoms?

Hot flushes are waves of heat rising within the body. Fresh air is beneficial in this case. As ovulation occurs less often, and eventually ceases altogether, a woman may become irritable and tired, or even have fits of depression and heart pains or outbreaks of sweating, and a tendency to put on weight.

What is the cause?

Ovulation begins at about twelve to fourteen and is followed by regular monthly periods, which then cease between the ages of forty-eight and fifty-two. Hormones continue to be produced, but not to the same extent as before, and this leads to the complaints described above. In severe cases, the doctor will prescribe extra hormones, in tablet form. In addition a course of acupressure, in consultation with a doctor, will improve the situation.

Body acupressure

The key point of the menopause is the *shang-chiao,* which lies in the first hollow of the sacrum, the central bone of the pelvis. Massage it downwards. Next, there is the *ming-men* ('gateway of life') point, situated between the second and third lumbar vertebrae, which should be massaged upwards. You will probably need someone else to massage these points for you.

The stimulus point for the heart and psyche,

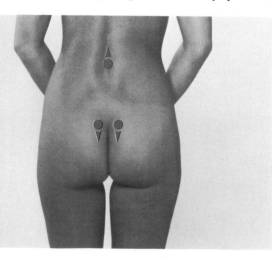

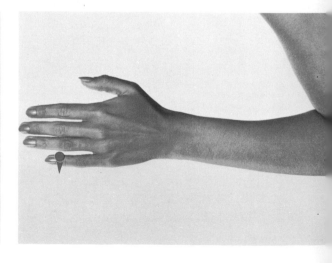

the *shao-chong,* lying near the inside lower corner of the little fingernail, should be massaged, across the finger, just below the nail, from the inside out. Finally, you can also massage the *tung-li* point, on the inner arm, two finger-widths above the base of the palm, on an imaginary line extended from the little finger. Massage it towards the little finger.

Ear acupressure

On the right ear, find the points for the ovaries and the womb, in the channel within the ridge of the ear where it emerges from the central hollow, and massage them well towards the top of the ear. Next, the points associated with hormone secretion from the pituitary gland, at the bottom of the central hollow, should be massaged upwards and backwards. On the left ear, reverse the directions.

Treatment

Ear and body acupressure should be alternated daily, for periods of five to ten minutes a day. With improvement, it may be possible to reduce the hormone treatment prescribed by your doctor, but only in consultation with him. In cases of the so-called 'male menopause', the same points should be used.

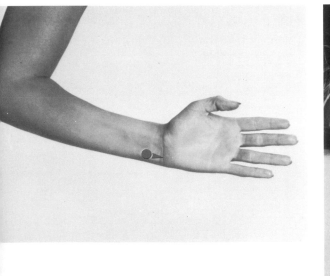

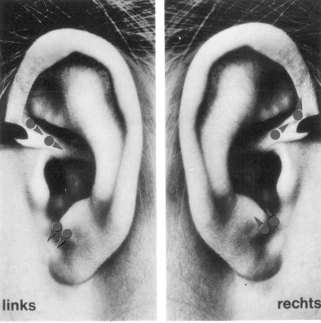

links   rechts

Keeping fit

Too much stress often gives rise to a lack of energy and a general feeling of fatigue. People should use acupressure to keep fit as habitually as they drink tea or coffee during work breaks. Deep-seated causes of fatigue can only be excluded by a medical examination.

How to recognize a lack of energy

It may start by friends at work saying you need a holiday. Then you yourself realize that you haven't got things under control. When this happens, give yourself a course of acupressure on the fitness points.

What are the causes?

Fatigue is usually due to overwork and too much pressure. Sometimes, psychological problems such as frustration may play a part. A previous illness may have the same effect.

Body acupressure

The heart and psyche are stimulated through the *shao-chong* ('heart of a wave') point, on the inside of the little finger of the left hand, beside the nail. Massage the finger, below the nail, from the inside out.

Next, there is the *ho-ku* point, two finger-widths below the knuckle of the forefinger, and half a finger-width towards the thumb, which should be massaged towards the elbow. This is particularly useful if you are exhausted from over-exertion.

The main point for all kinds of physical weakness is the *lieh-ch'üeh* ('past the straits'), which lies on the inside of the arm, two finger-widths above the palm, at the point where the pulse is usually taken. Massage towards the thumb.

People sometimes get exhausted from a combination of nervousness and being rushed, instead of being able to take things in their turn. In this case, the *tsu-san-li* ('asiatic peace' or 'heavenly calm') point gives relief. You find it by placing the palm of your hand on your kneecap, so that your middle finger reaches your shin; the point then lies directly beneath the tip of the fourth finger, and should be massaged downwards.

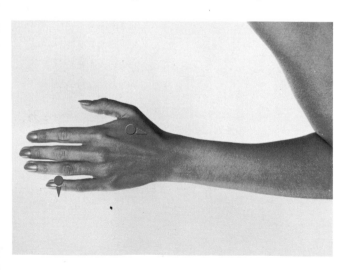

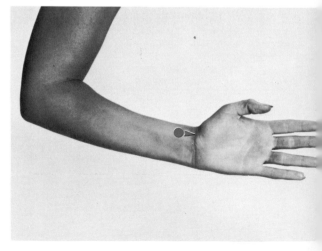

Ear acupressure

'Energy-giving' massage should be carried out on both ears. This has the effect of stimulating the hormones and relieving nervous tension. On the right ear, the ridge around the central hollow is massaged from top to bottom. The nerve-stimulation point on the front ridge, where it emerges from the central hollow, should be massaged forwards and upwards, and the whole of the front part of the ear, near where it joins the head, should be massaged upwards. Reverse the directions for the left ear.

A word of advice

It is not always wise to use acupressure to generate extra energy. Before doing so, give some thought to getting a proper night's sleep and abstaining from alcohol and tobacco, especially if you are under pressure. Try to relax at weekends and on holiday, and try to get a change of scene for a holiday, too.

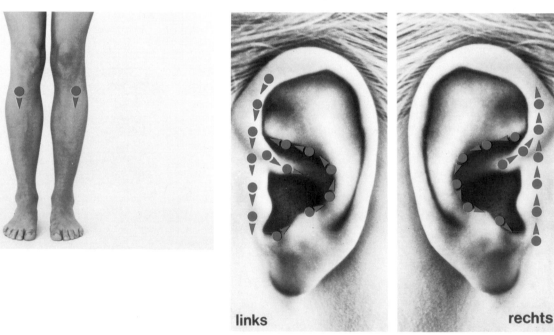

links   rechts

93

Kidney malfunction

Nowadays we hear a lot about artificial kidneys and kidney transplants, but these are the last resort in very severe cases, where all other treatment has failed. Ideally, no one should reach this stage, since even after a serious illness the kidneys are capable of becoming sound and functioning normally again. Acupressure is beneficial in two ways: in helping to restore the kidneys after an illness, or in strengthening them on a day-to-day basis.

What are the symptoms of a poorly functioning kidney?

If your urine becomes cloudy, see your doctor straightaway. If a kidney is diseased, it will show up in a simple chemical test, and the doctor will diagnose the exact nature of the complaint. Another sign is persistent back pains, which is commonly put down to disc trouble, but which may also be due to kidney disease.

What are the causes?

The kidneys are the body's waste-disposal unit. They can be damaged by what can only be described as poisons taken over a long period, such as Phenacetin, or inflamed by exposure to cold, possibly just by following the fashion for exposing one's midriff! A badly inflamed bladder may eventually affect the kidneys as well. All such cases must be treated by a doctor, but sometimes even the best treatment fails to cure the inflammation completely. However, if at the onset of the complaint you combine acupressure with expert medical treatment, you have a much better chance of being permanently cured.

Body acupressure

The first point, the *t'ai-hsi,* lies just below and behind the inner anklebone, in a little hollow, and should be massaged downwards and backwards. Next, the *yin-ku* point should be massaged upwards. This point will be found, with the knee bent, at the inner end of the crease in a hollow between two tendons. Another important point affecting the kidneys is the *ching-men,* also known as the 'energy point of consent'. This is situated at the open end of the twelfth rib, and is easily found if you stand up

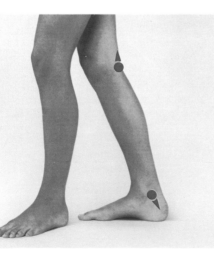

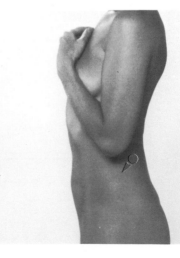

and place your bent arm on your body, measuring four finger-widths back from the point of the elbow. Massage it forwards and downwards. In combination with this, massage the *shen-shu* point (the 'point of equilibrium of the kidneys') in a downward direction. This lies two to three finger-widths to each side of the base of the second lumbar vertebra.

Ear acupressure

The 'kidney point' lies within the fold of the upper edge of the ear, where it begins to curve towards the back of the head. Starting at this point, massage right into the fold, first upwards, then backwards. The central energy point, on the ridge, where it emerges from the central hollow, should also be massaged, forwards and upwards. Reverse the directions on the left ear.

Treatment

Ear and body acupressure should be alternated daily, one to three times a day, for five to ten minutes, for average disorders. If you have been prescribed any drugs or medicines, keep taking them. When tests show that the kidneys are functioning normally again, you can gradually reduce the treatment, and then just do it once or twice a week.

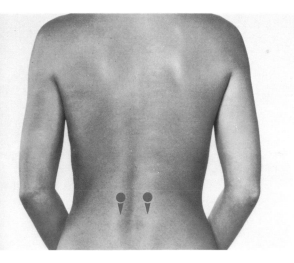

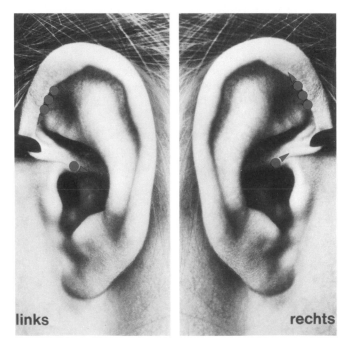

links   rechts

95

Knee pains

Knee pains are particularly common among overweight people and the elderly. As you walk, you put practically all your body-weight on the knee joints which, when overloaded, start to give pain.

What are the symptoms?

The pains are felt in the general area of the knee, extending down in the lower leg. There is often a swelling around the knee joint as well.

What is the cause?

Inside the knee joint there are two menisci, an outer and an inner one. They are lens-shaped discs which prevent friction and ensure a good fit at the joint between the thighbone and the lower legbone. At the ends of the bones there is the usual layer of cartilage which, like the menisci, is subject to wear. In an advanced stage, this is called arthrosis of the knee; if the joint becomes inflamed, it is called arthritis. In both cases, the doctor will prescribe medicines, and sometimes give injections direct into the joint itself. While acupressure cannot reverse the wearing process on the joint, it can nevertheless relieve the pain and prevent, or slow down, any worsening of the condition.

Body acupressure

The first point, *tsu-san-li,* is found by placing the palm of the hand on the kneecap, so that the middle finger touches the shin: it then lies immediately beneath the tip of the ring finger. Just above it, and to the side, directly in front of and below the top of the outer legbone, lies the *yang-ling-ch'üan* point. Massage both points downwards. The *nei-chung* point, at the centre of the fold of the knee, should also be massaged downwards. There are also four local points, situated above and below, and on each side of the knee. These should be massaged away from the knee.

Ear acupressure

Even if only one knee is affected, you should massage both ears and the points on both sides of the body, but press more firmly on the affected side. On the ear, the 'knee point' lies in

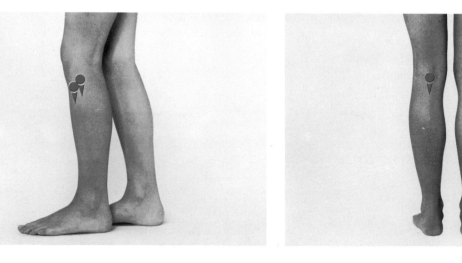

the centre of the small, triangular hollow above the central ridge. Massage it upwards and forwards on the right ear. Though not illustrated, the equivalent point on the back of the ear should also be massaged, this time downwards. The main energy point is situated on the central ridge, where it emerges from the central hollow; massage it firmly in an upward direction. Reverse the directions of massage on the left ear.

Treatment

Ear and body acupressure should be alternated daily. The length and frequency of treatment depend on the severity of the complaint, and will vary from once to three times a day, for five to ten minutes at a time. As soon as your condition improves you may be able to reduce your intake of drugs, but only in consultation with your doctor.

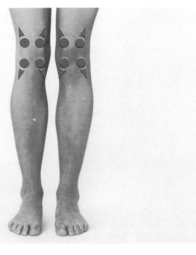

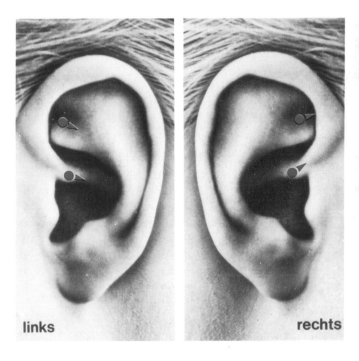

links   rechts

Liver trouble

The liver could be called the body's 'chemical factory'. It breaks up the food particles, absorbed by the intestinal wall, and turns them into energy-giving and body-building substances; it also removes the poisons from the system. It needs to function properly for the sake of our energy store and general well-being but, regrettably, we often overload it, usually by drinking too much alcohol. The liver has one peculiarity, which can be fatal: it does not immediately warn us when it is overloaded. If you start to feel a dull pain under the right rib cage, spreading across the back, you already have some form of liver complaint.

What are the signs of a poorly functioning liver?

A deep-seated liver complaint is usually preceded by a persistent feeling of fatigue, but it is of such a general nature that there is no obvious connection with the liver. However, if your stools become pale in colour, and your urine brown, you have the systems of an inflamed liver, and should *see your doctor straightaway*. He will probably make chemical tests of the liver processes, and, if they are abnormal, put you on a diet and prescribe appropriate drugs. If you combine these with acupressure you will soon be strong and well again.

What are the causes?

Every time you overload your liver, you damage it, especially if poisons are present, which the liver has to deal with. One of the worst of these is alcohol: if your doctor confirms that you have a liver complaint you *must* abstain *completely,* until your liver is restored and the doctor allows you to drink in moderation again. Acupressure does *not* exempt you from the ban on alcohol.

Body acupressure

First, the *t'ai-chung* point, two to three finger-widths above the crease between the big and second toes, and slightly towards the former, should be massaged upwards. Next, the *tchong-tu* point, one finger-width below and to the rear of, the halfway mark on an imaginary line between the centre of the kneecap and the

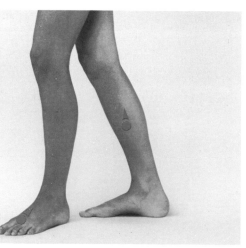

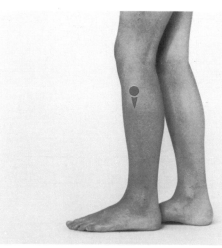

inner anklebone. Massage it upwards. There is an important point three finger-widths below the top of the fibula (outer legbone), which should be massaged strongly in a downward direction. Lastly, the points *ion-trang,* halfway up the breastbone, and *tan-chung,* two finger-widths lower down, should be massaged upwards.

Ear acupressure

As the liver lies mainly on the right side of the body, you need only massage the right ear to affect it directly. Your 'organ point', in the central hollow, should be massaged upwards.

The point of supply for the nerves, which is on the upper rim of the central hollow, should be massaged strongly downwards and backwards. The central 'energy point', at the start of the central ridge, should be massaged upwards. This is the only point on the left ear to be massaged; reverse the direction.

Treatment

The liver is an organ which repairs itself very well. Ear and body acupressure should be alternated daily, one to three times a day, for five to ten minutes, depending on the severity of the complaint.

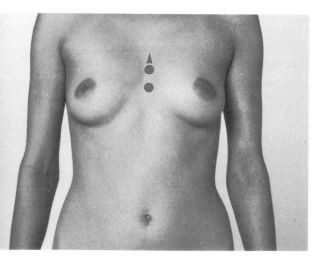

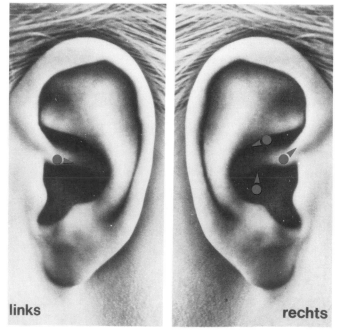

links   rechts

Migraine

1 Migraine caused by an upset liver or gall bladder, localized behind and around one of the eyes

This is the commonest form of migraine, so will be dealt with first in this six-part section.

What are the symptoms?

This type of migraine begins as a headache behind one eye, which then develops into a continuous, piercing pain on one side of the head. It frequently starts in the small hours, so you go to bed with a clear head and wake up in severe pain.

What are the causes?

According to the Chinese, the so-called 'gall meridian' lies close to the eye and leads directly into it. When specifically questioned, many patients who suffer from a piercing pain behind the eye also admit to feeling discomfort under the right rib cage, and, if the condition persists for several days, it is also common for the patient's stools to become lighter in colour than normal.

Migraine is frequently brought on by alcohol, eggs, chocolate, fatty pork, and even coffee, if it has not been properly filtered after roasting. All these foods are bad for the liver and gall bladder in any case, and if there is tension in the bile ducts, including those of the liver, they can trigger an attack. Patients suffer from malfunction of the gall bladder and, in many cases, from constipation.

Migraine may also be due to psychological causes. Traditionally, the gall bladder is the seat of the temperament and if there is tension in the bile ducts, it only needs excitement or agitation for an onset to occur. The liver and gall bladder function together, with the result that certain liver complaints are a further cause. This form of migraine is very difficult to diagnose, particularly since tension in the bile ducts does not always show up on X-rays.

Body acupressure

The central point for treating tension in the bile ducts lies three finger-widths below the top of

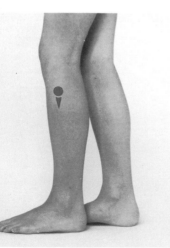 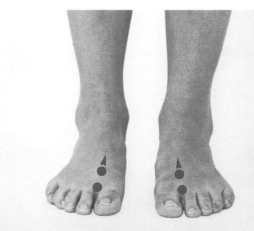

100

the fibula (outer legbone). This should be massaged downwards. The other points are the *hsing-chien,* in the crease between the big toe and the second toe, and the *t'ai-ch'ung,* two to three finger-widths higher up. Massage both upwards. Localized points of pain in the head should be softly rubbed with the fingers, upwards, downwards and sideways, as shown.

Ear acupressure

As a general rule, acupressure should only be applied to the right ear, even if the pain is felt on the left side, or on both sides. In most cases, migraine occurs on the right side. The points for the gall bladder and liver are all situated in the hollow of the ear, and should be massaged around the ridge. The 'motor-point' for the gall bladder is found in the hollow behind the ear and should be massaged downwards.

Treatment

Ear and body acupressure should be alternated daily, one to three times a day, for periods of five to ten minutes. A suitable diet should also be followed, supplemented, if necessary, by veget-able-based medicines prescribed by your doctor, to stimulate the functions of the liver and gall bladder.

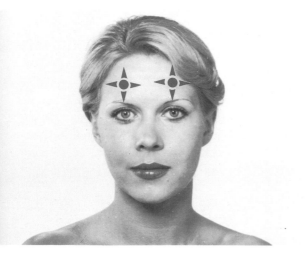

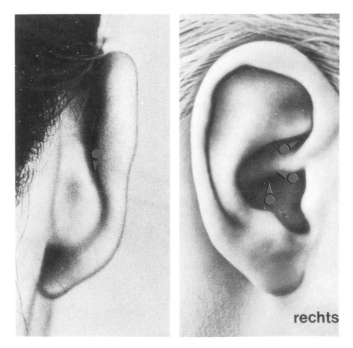

rechts

101

Migraine

2 Migraine caused by the weather affecting the head generally, and often just the forehead

This form of migraine is widespread in areas which are subject to marked changes of climate.

What are the symptoms?

With some patients the headache begins *before* a change in the weather, in others it occurs *afterwards*. In both cases, the effect of the weather is to blame.

What is the cause?

Doctors do not know why body functions should be affected by the weather, but that they are is shown by the fact that sufferers have fewer headaches in an area with a constant climate, such as a holiday resort. However, this is not necessarily conclusive since people are not usually under stress on holiday.

If in doubt yourself, consult an experienced acupuncturist. You may *sense* more causes for your headaches than there really are and, unfortunately, the same are present in migraines with multiple causes. If this applies in your case, combine the appropriate courses of acupressure, massaging all the ear points on one day and all the body points on the next, and so on.

Body acupressure

The important point is the one which stimulates all the body functions at once. Called the *chung-chu,* it is situated on the back of the hand, one finger below the knuckle of the ring finger, and half a finger-width towards the little finger. Massage it firmly towards the elbow.

The second point is *szu-chu-k'ung,* at the outer end of each eyebrow; massage it downwards to a point one finger-width from the outer corner of the eye.

Finally, there are the three points, *chung-kuan,* halfway between the base of the breastbone and the navel, *cha-iuenn,* three to four finger-widths lower down, and *shang-kuan,* two finger-widths above the first point. Massage all three in an upward direction.

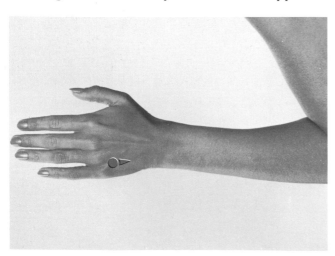

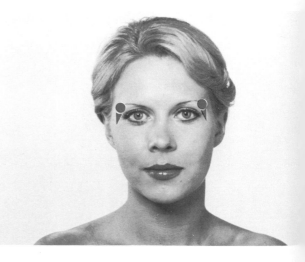

Ear acupressure

On the right ear, the 'weather points' should be massaged strongly upwards. They extend from the start of the central ridge to the face. There is a central 'nerve point' at the foot of the central hollow, and another point on the face, just in front of the upper edge of the lobe, both of which should be massaged upwards. On the left ear, reverse the directions of massage for all points.

Treatment

Ear and body acupressure should be alternated daily. If, to start with, you find that this brings on more headaches, rub the local areas of pain on the head gently with the finger, upwards, downwards, and to each side.

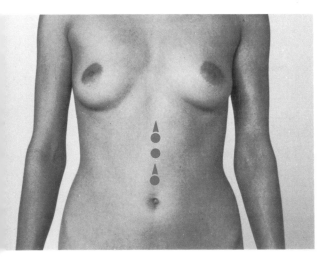

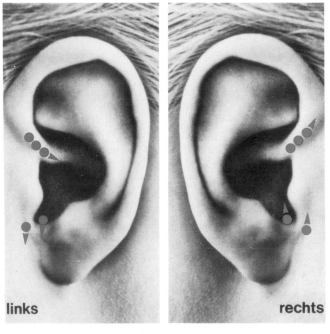

links   rechts

Migraine

3 Migraine due to hormonal imbalance, usually starting at the temples, then spreading to the forehead and eventually to the whole head

According to acupuncturists, this type of headache or migraine is the third most common. It is put down to a hormone imbalance between the oestrogens and the progestogens.

What are the symptoms?

The direct connection between periods of hormonal activity and migraine attacks is most obvious during the early stages of the illness; later it is less clear. Some patients start having attacks, in the form of headaches, at the time of their first period, when they are twelve to fourteen years old. After that, the headaches come on shortly before a period, and sometimes midway between periods as well, during ovulation.

You can tell this type of migraine from the fact that, during pregnancy, at the latest after the sixth to eighth month, migraine attacks disappear completely, only to return again, as badly as ever soon after the birth of the child. In women with several children, this association is often quite striking. If a woman gets attacks with increasing frequency (and some have them every other day), the connection with hormonal activity is less obvious. In this case, it may help to go back to the very beginning of the illness to establish the cause.

What is the cause?

During the monthly cycle, two hormones are produced, oestradiol and progesterone. Migraine is not so much due to the amount secreted as to an imbalance between the two. As a rule, the cause is too little oestradiol and too much progesterone, and certain kinds of contraceptive pill, which are based on this imbalance, may lead to migraine. There is also an illness, called endometriosis, which may have the same effect. If you suspect that your migraine is due to hormonal causes, see your gynecologist, and an experienced acupuncturist.

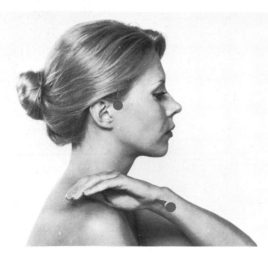

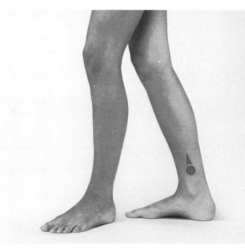

Body acupressure

The first point is the *k'o-chu-jen,* two finger-widths in front of the ear, in a hollow which is evident when you open your mouth. Massage it upwards. Next, the *tung-li* point, two or three finger-widths above the inside edge of the wrist, on a line extended from the little finger, should be massaged towards the little finger.

Two further points, the *san-yin-chiao,* three to four finger-widths above the point of the inner anklebone, on the edge of the shin, and the *ch'i-hai* (not illustrated), two to three finger-widths (four to five, if you are fat) below the navel, should both be massaged upwards. Finally, the principal hormone point, the *shang-chiao,* which lies in the first hollow of the sacrum (central bone of the pelvis), should be massaged downwards.

Ear acupressure

The points for the ovaries and the uterus lie in the channel in the rising ridge of the ear. Massage them upwards on the right ear. The 'hormone control points', at the bottom and on the edge of the central hollow, should be massaged upwards and backwards, on the right ear. Reverse the directions on the left ear.

Treatment

Ear and body acupressure should be alternated daily. Massage strongly on days before an expected attack, which usually means just before a period is due. If your doctor has prescribed treatment with hormones or a change of contraceptive pill, you must continue with it.

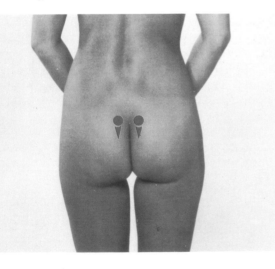

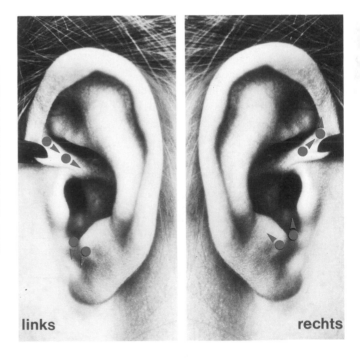

links   rechts

Migraine

4 Migraine due to spinal causes, starting at the top of the spine and spreading forwards

This is another common form of the complaint, known to doctors as 'cervical migraine'.

What are the symptoms?

As a rule, this form of migraine comes on in later life, when any damage to the upper spine starts to show, but there are exceptions where, for instance, people have been involved in an accident of some sort. The headache starts in the upper part of the spine (cervical vertebrae) and spreads forwards.

What are the causes?

There are two basic causes, both of which may unfortunately be present. The chief reason is a damaged disc in the region of the fifth, sixth or seventh cervical vertebra. This irritates the nerve ends and sets up tension in the spinal column, which spreads upwards and brings on a headache. An X-ray will show whether this is the cause.

The other reason is that the upper spine may have shifted and twisted slightly, affecting the first, sixth, and seventh cervical vertebrae in particular. There are doctors who specialize in relocating displaced vertebrae, and you should consult one of these. At the same time, take a course of acupressure (and, in a severe case, acupuncture as well) to avoid a recurrence of the complaint.

Body acupressure

The first points are the *t'ien-chu*, which lies two finger-widths to the side of the centre line of the neck, just above the hairline; the *ta-chu*, two finger-widths to the side of the prominent first dorsal vertebra; and another point (not illustrated) which is very sensitive to pressure, and which lies exactly halfway between the previous two. Massage all these points downwards. The *ta-chui* point, which is just below the bulge of the seventh cervical vertebra, should be massaged upwards.

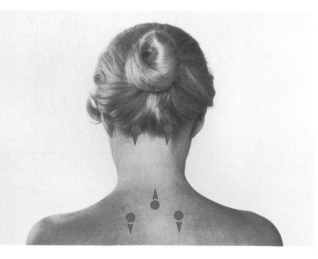

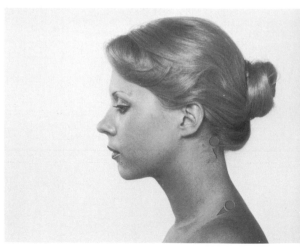

Next, there are the points *fung-ch'ih,* three finger-widths back from the base of the ear, behind the projecting bone and just beyond the hair line, and *chien-ching,* one hand-width below the previous point, on the highest part of the shoulder (where the shoulder meets the neck). Massage both points downwards.

Finally, the *t'suan-chu* point, at the inner end of each eyebrow, should be massaged upwards. Any localized areas of pain at the back of the head should be rubbed gently with the finger, upwards, downwards, and to each side.

Ear acupressure

On the right ear, massage the points for the upper spine, around the central hollow, in an upward direction, as well as the central 'energy point' at the start of the ridge, and another point at the lower front of the lobe. All the points on the left ear should be massaged downwards. Apply more pressure on the side which gives most pain.

Treatment

Ear and body acupressure should be alternated daily, once to three times a day, for five to ten minutes, depending on the severity of the complaint. As a rule, it is better to keep the head still and let the headache pass than to apply strong massage.

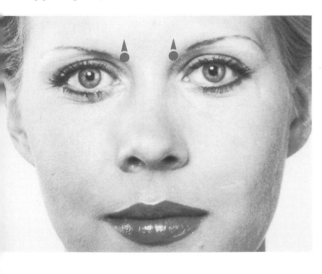

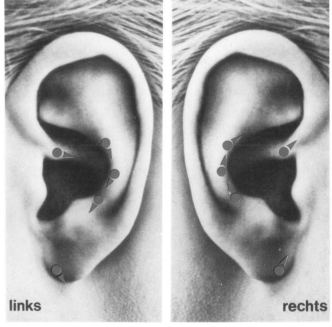

links   rechts

Migraine

5 Migraine due to a depressed state of mind, with no particular localization

What are the symptoms?

Depressions frequently cause tension in the muscles near the spine, especially in the neck, leading to a general headache in the forehead and temples. It is important to distinguish between this type and the headache caused by damage to the cervical vertebrae. With depression-based migraine, the tension in the neck is not so pronounced.

What is the cause?

Depression can take on a variety of symptoms, such as disturbed nights, headaches and heart pains, especially at the start, before the actual, depressed state of mind shows itself. Of all the symptoms, headaches are among the most common. A clear sign of this form of migraine is that none of the usual headache pills or powders does any good. The only way to relieve the headache is to treat the cause, the depression itself. (For details of the causes of depression, see the section on page 52).

Acupressure

It must be repeated that only the treatment of the depression is worthwhile, so apply acupressure as described on pages 52 and 53. However, you can also relieve localized points of pain by rubbing them carefully with the finger, upwards, downwards and to each side. The illustration shows the *tae yang* point which is a common point of pain.

Treatment

As described on page 53.

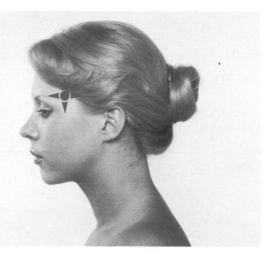

Migraine

6 Migraine or headaches due to other causes

The most common causes of headaches have been described in the previous sections, but these are by no means the only ones. Why should there be so many? Quite simply, the body has only a limited number of ways of giving us information. In your car, you have warning lights to tell you if anything goes wrong, but the body has no such system. Its main alarm signal is pain, and it uses this to draw our attention to an illness which needs to be cured. Throughout this book, I have dealt with the cause of every complaint, and it is this, rather than the mere removing of the symptoms, which is the subject of the treatment described. Now to other causes of headaches.

You may get a headache in the forehead, as a result of eye strain. These 'ophthalmic' migraines can usually be cured, either by starting to wear glasses, or getting a stronger pair, so if you think you are suffering from ophthalmic migraine, have your eyes tested as soon as possible. If eye strain is confirmed by your oculist, apply acupressure as shown in the accompanying illustration. And don't forget to make sure that your desk is properly lit.

A medical examination may be needed to diagnose the types of headache described hitherto, but it is absolutely vital to have one if there is any suspicion that the headaches might be caused by a brain tumour or other form of brain disease. There is no place for acupressure in such cases as these. Acupressure is very beneficial when it is properly used on the right illness. But let your doctor decide whether your illness is suitable for acupressure treatment.

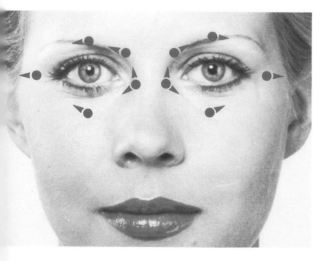

Mouth, inflammation of the lining

This can occur as a straightforward inflammation, due to some local irritation (from tartar deposits, false teeth, inflamed gums, or poor mouth care), or as a symptom of a serious illness, usually some sort of fever.

What are the symptoms?

The mouth lining is red and swollen and tends to bleed. Sometimes it gets coated as well. You find it difficult to eat and, if the inflammation is bad, even to speak.

What is the cause?

It usually accompanies inflammation of the gums due to a lack of proper mouth care. Ulcers and signs of severe inflammation are symptoms of a more serious illness, and in this case it would be wrong to use acupressure to treat the symptoms alone. You must have proper medical treatment for the illness itself, but you can also use acupressure, in consultation with your doctor, to reduce the inflammation.

Body acupressure

There are two points for the mucous membranes: the first, the *ho-ku,* is two finger-widths below the knuckle of the fore finger and half a finger-width towards the thumb. The second, the *hou-hsi,* lies just below, and towards the outside edge of the knuckle of the little finger. Massage both points in the direction of the elbow. The *ch'eng-chiang* point has a more local effect: it lies in the crease in the centre of the lower lip, and should be massaged upwards.

Ear acupressure

On the right ear, the points on the lobe relating to the mouth and gums should be massaged upwards and backwards. There is also the general energy point, on the ridge where it emerges from the central hollow, which should be massaged upwards and forwards. Reverse the direction of massage on the left ear.

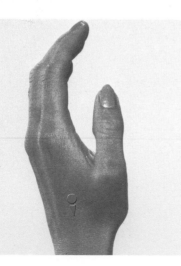

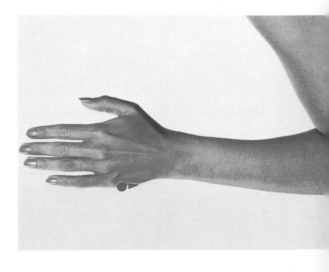

Treatment

Ear and body acupressure should be alternated daily, one to three times a day, depending on the severity of the complaint. You should also have camomile mouthwashes (in China they tend to use herbal remedies in conjunction with acupressure).

If your case is simply due to tartar deposits or an ill-fitting denture, see your dentist as soon as possible. However, if the inflammation is a symptom of a serious illness, you must of course call in the doctor. In both cases, acupressure acts as a complementary form of treatment, nothing more.

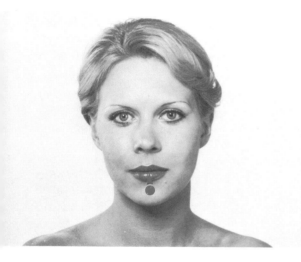

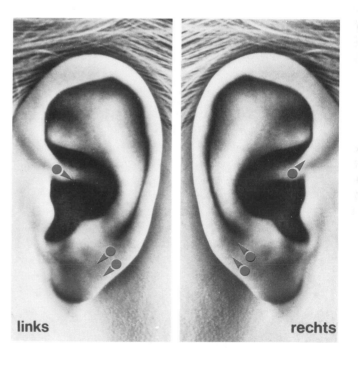

links   rechts

Nausea, travelsickness and early morning sickness

As a body function, these three complaints go together, originating from an upset in the nervous system of the throat and stomach. You will find that acupressure gives welcome relief in cases of frequent travel or early-morning sickness. However, if you have an upset stomach from eating and drinking too much, or from the wrong kind of food, you should not try to prevent vomiting by acupressure, but should bring it on instead, by putting your finger down your throat. This will relieve the feeling of nausea, and you will soon feel well again.

What are the symptoms?

First there is a feeling of nausea, often followed by vomiting, especially when travelling by sea.

What are the causes?

Travel sickness is usually due to a disturbance of the balance mechanism when it is unable to find fixed reference points. Like early-morning sickness, which is due to hormonal and psychological causes, it seems to be a question of habit. In general, however, the more children a woman has, the less she suffers from this complaint. If nausea is felt more or less continuously, as is the case with kidney or liver disease, you should get your doctor to give you a thorough examination, and then apply acupressure in consultation with him.

Body acupressure

The *chang-men* point should be massaged forwards and upwards. You will find it on the side of the body, immediately below the point of the elbow, when the patient is standing with his arm bent against the side of his body.

Next, the *ch'i men* point, which lies on a direct line below the nipple and two finger-widths below the projecting breastbone, between the sixth and seventh ribs, should be massaged upwards.

The *liang-men* point, which is directly linked

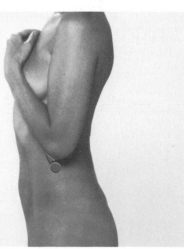

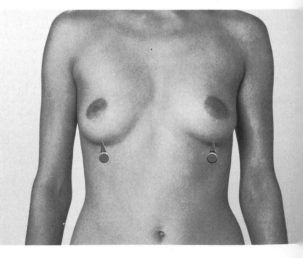

to the stomach, five to six finger-widths above and three finger-widths to the side of the navel, should be massaged downwards.

Finally, there is the general energy point, the *chi-hai,* which is two to three (on fat people, four to five) finger-widths below the navel. Massage it upwards.

Ear acupressure

There are several points in the hollow on the back of the ear, half a finger-width from the edge, which correspond to the throat and stomach, and these should be massaged upwards. On the front of the ear at the base of the ridge emerging from the central hollow,

there are other points which should be massaged in a clockwise direction. The main nerve point for the stomach and abdomen, on the ridge itself, should be massaged forwards and upwards. Generally speaking, acupressure is not applied to the left ear in this case.

Treatment

For travel sickness it is better to treat just the ear points. In cases of prolonged early-morning sickness, and after consultation with your doctor, apply ear and body acupressure on alternate days, early in the morning and, if necessary, half an hour before meals as well, for five to ten minutes at a time.

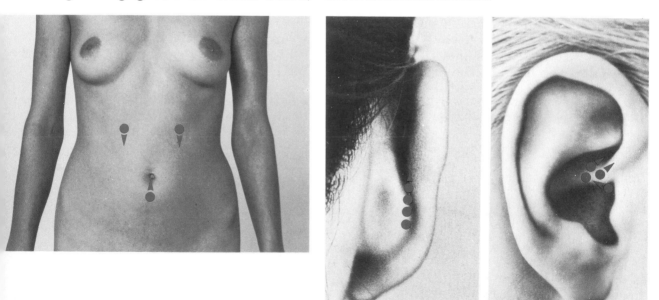

rechts

113

Nervousness and irritability

Nervousness is so widespread nowadays that people have almost come to regard it as normal. Even on holiday, many of us are still nervous and irritable, so we fail to recover our mental poise before we return to the daily round.

What are the symptoms?

It is sometimes almost impossible to talk to someone in this state. This is where acupressure is very beneficial but it may not be easy to get the message across to the other person that he needs to try it.

What are the causes?

You can only live in harmony with yourself when you can offset periods of activity with periods of rest. This is the point of sleep and of restful weekends and holidays, but if these too are subject to stress and rushing about, you get nervous and irritable. Acupressure cannot replace your need for rest and relaxation but it can help you to get things in proportion again.

Body acupressure

As main points you take the 'chin point' *pai-hui*, which lies in the middle of the skull on an imaginary line joining the tops of your ears, and the *hou-ting*, which lies in a small but obvious hollow about three finger widths behind it. Massage both points forwards. In addition, the *chin-wei* point at the base of the breastbone should be massaged upwards. The fourth point in the combination is *tsu-san-li*, on the lower leg, which you will find beneath the tip of your ring finger if you put the palm of your hand on your kneecap; this should be massaged downwards.

Ear acupressure

On the right ear there are two important 'brain points': the first lies on the lobe, just below the central hollow, and should be massaged downwards; the second, in front of the first and slightly higher up, should be massaged upwards. The central energy point, on the ridge where it emerges from the central hollow,

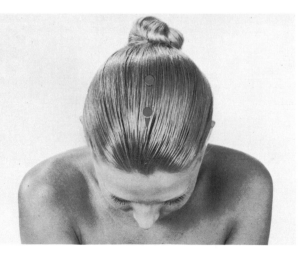

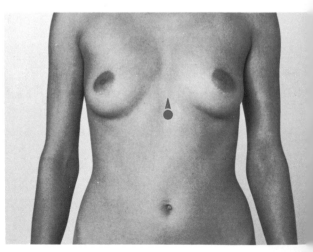

should be massaged forwards and upwards. Massage the points on the left ear in the opposite direction.

Treatment

Ear and body acupressure should be alternated daily, from one to three times a day, for five to ten minutes, depending on the degree of nervousness and irritability displayed. Periods of rest and sound sleep are essential.

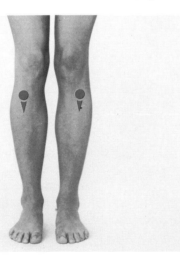

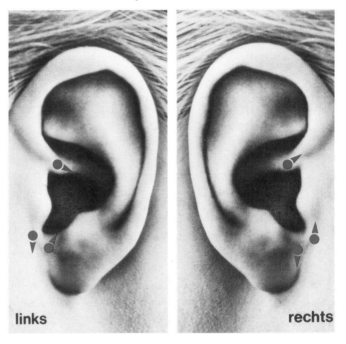

links   rechts

Nosebleeds

Nosebleeds are common among children, but should only occur occasionally. They are sometimes caused simply by scratching the inside of the nostril with a sharp fingernail. As an illness, bleeding occurs frequently and heavily, or it may be linked to another, possibly serious, complaint.

What are the symptoms?

The fine veins in the lining of the nose rupture and bleed. Very occasionally there may be heavy bleeding, in which case the doctor will pack the nostril with gauze.

What is the cause?

What usually happens with children is that the lining of the nose gets dry, and then they scratch inside the nostril with their fingernail. Acupressure is useful in such cases to strengthen the inner membrane. An accident resulting in a fractured nose or skull would be another cause. Finally, nosebleeds can be a sign of something more serious, such as high blood pressure, heart disease, blood congestion, a blood clot (thrombosis), or some form of infectious disease. If you suspect any of these, see your doctor immediately.

Body acupressure

The main point for the lining of the nose is the *ho-ku,* two finger-widths below the index finger knuckle and half a finger-width towards the thumb. Massage it in the direction of the elbow. The second point is the *mi-tchong,* on the hairline, one and a half finger-widths from the middle of the forehead. Massage it outwards.

The relaxation point, the *tsu-san-li,* should be massaged downwards. This point is on the lower leg, directly beneath the tip of your ring finger when you put the palm of your hand on your kneecap. The last two points are *hsing-chien,* which is in the crease between the big and second toe, but nearer the big toe; and *t'ai-chung,* which is two to three finger-widths higher up. Both should be massaged towards the ankle.

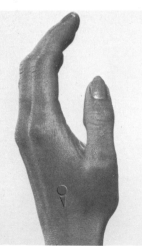

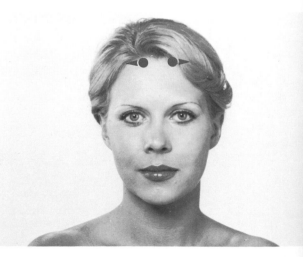

Ear acupressure

On the right ear, the 'nose point', which is at the lower, front edge of the lobe, should be massaged upwards. The 'central energy point', which is on the ridge where it emerges from the central hollow, should also be massaged upwards. Reverse the directions of massage on the left ear.

Treatment

Ear and body acupressure should be alternated daily. In the acute stage, concentrate more on ear acupressure. You can also rub a suitable ointment into the nostrils, making sure that it penetrates as far up as possible by holding the nose gently and breathing in at the same time.

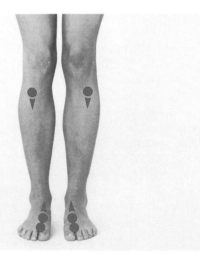

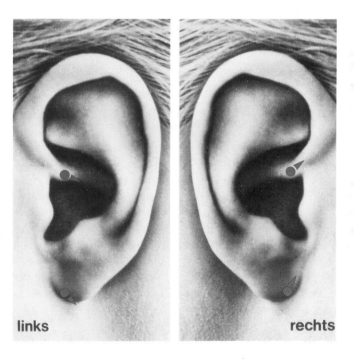

links   rechts

An 'over-full' feeling

As this is a sign of illness or of a functional defect, it is important to start by finding out exactly where the root cause lies. Although it is commonly mentioned by patients as a symptom, it is not usually put down to overeating. What we understand by the term here is the feeling which is brought on by only a small meal, and which then remains for some time afterwards.

What are the symptoms?

Quite simply, you feel 'blown out' after every meal.

What are the causes?

The defect lies somewhere in the area of the tube connecting the stomach to the intestine. Any one of a number of factors may be involved, such as a weakness in the stomach's digestive system, or in the liver or gall-bladder. It may be that the pancreas is not functioning properly, or that the intestine itself is contributing to the feeling, through sluggishness or tension. There may even be a more general deficiency. There are so many possibilities that it needs a doctor to isolate the problem in each particular case, and acupressure should only be practised in consultation with him.

Body acupressure

Beginning with the foot, the stimulus point for the pancreas, the *ta-tu*, should be massaged towards the heel. This point is situated on the inside of the big toe, just in front of the ball of the foot, where the colour of the skin changes from pink to white. Combine this with the *chieh-hsi* point, the stimulus point of the stomach, which lies in the centre of the angle joint, at the base of the shinbone, in a noticeable hollow between two tendons; massage it downwards.

Next, the *san-yin-chiao* point, two to three finger-widths above the inner anklebone, at the back edge of the shinbone, should be massaged upwards. The *tchong-tu* point, one finger-width backwards and down from a point midway between the centre of the kneecap and the inner anklebone, should also be massaged upwards. The important point for the gall bladder is the *dang-nang-dian*, three finger-widths below the

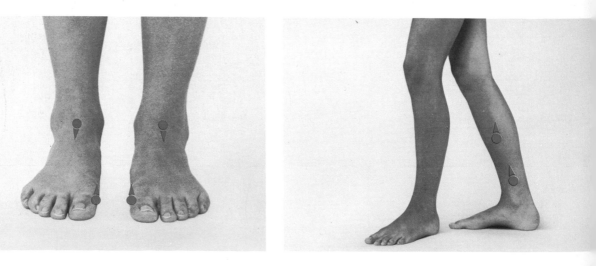

head of the outer legbone (fibula), and this should be massaged firmly, in a downward direction.

Ear acupressure

On the right ear, the points in the central hollow associated with the liver, gall bladder, and pancreas should be massaged upwards. The central point for all abdominal activity, the 'point of the solar plexus', must be massaged as strongly as possible in an upward direction. This point lies on the central ridge where it emerges from the central hollow. As a rule, treatment of the right ear is sufficient, but you can also massage the solar-plexus point on the left ear if

you wish – massage it backwards and downwards.

Treatment

The acupressure described here will stimulate the functions of the stomach, gall bladder, liver, and pancreas. On the advice of your doctor you could also make use of the appropriate acupressure treatment for intestinal functions. Under normal circumstances, ear and body acupressure should be alternated daily. One treatment a day, lasting five to ten minutes, should be enough, but you can increase this to two or three times a day if you wish.

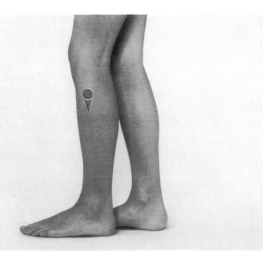

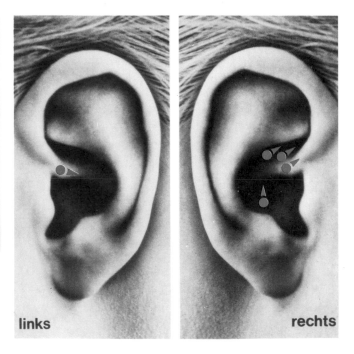

links   rechts

119

Pancreatic problems

In this case, acupressure should be regarded as a preventative measure, such as I have described in the introduction. It should be used, for example, on someone who has had severe pancreatitis, probably involving several weeks in hospital, and who is aware of the need to rest the pancreas by careful dieting and generally taking things easy. Acupressure in such cases can help to prevent a relapse.

What are the symptoms?

The pancreas performs the function of digesting food, which means breaking it down into its constituent parts (the human body produces one to one and a half litres of digestive juices a day). When the pancreas is not functioning properly the patient usually notices that something is wrong from the unusual nature and smell of his stools.

It goes without saying that acute inflammation of the pancreas, causing severe stomach pains, vomiting and circulatory failures should *never* be treated at home. *Immediate admission to hospital is essential.*

What are the causes?

The secretion of the digestive juices is controlled partly by the condition of the nervous vegetative system and partly by a hormone secreted by the duodenum, called secretin, so possible causes of pancreatic complaints may lie in the nervous vegetative system or in the small intestine. A stone in the pancreatic duct can also cause severe problems. In all cases you should have a medical examination, and only practise acupressure in consultation with your doctor.

Body acupressure

Apply acupressure to two points: the *kung-sun*, about one hand-width in front of the point of the inner anklebone, where the skin colour changes from pink to white; and the *san-yin-chiao*, four to five finger-widths above the point of the inner anklebone, at the back of the shinbone. Massage the former in the direction of the ankle-bone, and the latter upwards.

The 'inner barrier' point, which lies two to three finger-widths from the base of the palm, in

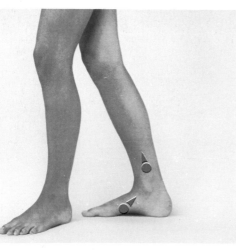 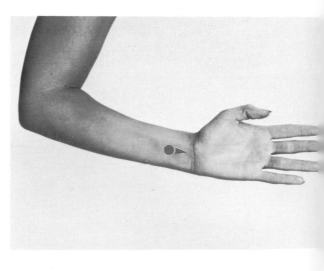

the centre of the inside arm, should also be massaged; in this case towards the hand. You should also get outside help to apply acupressure to the 'point of equilibrium' of the pancreas (Chinese name, *p'i-shu*), which is on the back, two to three finger-widths to the side of the lower edge of the eleventh vertebra. Massage it downwards.

Ear acupressure

As the pancreas lies across the abdomen, it has an appropriate point on each ear, both of which should receive treatment. The point lies in the upper hollow of the ear; on the right ear it

should be massaged towards the front, and on the left in the opposite direction.

Treatment

Carry out ear acupressure and body acupressure on alternate days, ideally half an hour before meals, for three to five minutes at a time. For minor cases, one treatment per day is enough, either in the morning or in the evening. As a preventative measure, one treatment a week is generally sufficient. Make sure that your doctor supervises your acupressure, and do not stop taking any drugs or medicines of your own accord.

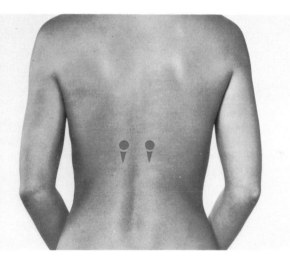

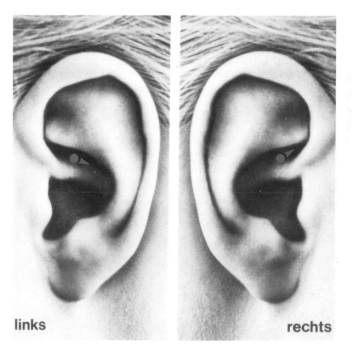

links   rechts

121

Phantom limb

Sometimes it is necessary to amputate an injured or diseased limb. It is not uncommon for the patient to feel racking pains in the limb which is no longer there, usually because the nerve concerned was injured or crushed when the accident took place. Many doctors believe that this impression of pain stays locked in the mind.

What are the symptoms?

The pains usually occur at night and the patient can quite often tell you the exact spot on the missing limb where the pain is at its worst.

What is the cause?

Medical opinion is divided on this subject. The Swiss doctor, Professor Kielholz, believes that phantom pains of this nature are comparable in many respects with depression. Some doctors think that the pains exist only in the mind and that the stump of the limb plays no part in the matter, while others hold the opposite view. Such differences of opinion are completely irrelevant as far as acupressure is concerned.

Body acupressure

You should apply the method known as 'pain-point acupressure' to the sound limb. For example, if the heel of the amputated left leg is giving pain, massage the heel of the remaining right leg vigorously. In principle, the direction of massage in such cases is upwards.

The general points requiring massage are the *pai-hui*, in the centre of the skull, on an imaginary line between the ears, and the *hou-ting*, about three finger-widths behind the first, in a noticeable hollow. Massage both points forwards. Next, the *ho-ku* point, which is two finger-widths below the centre of the knuckle of the index finger and half a finger-width towards the thumb, should be massaged in the direction of the elbow. Lastly, the *tsu-san-li* point should be massaged downwards. This lies on the lower leg, under the tip of your ring finger when you place the palm of your hand on your kneecap.

Ear acupressure

First, study the illustration and find the 'pain-point' on the right or left ear corresponding to

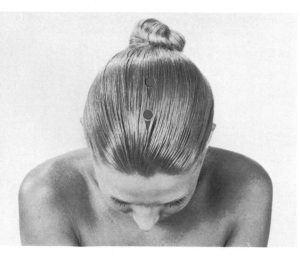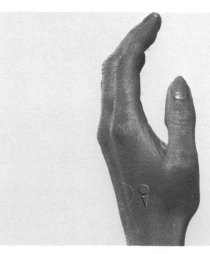

the missing limb, and massage it accordingly – upwards on the right ear, downwards on the left. There is also an important 'psychological point' for thought processes, at the bottom front of the ear lobe. Massage it firmly upwards.

Treatment

In these cases, the acupressure points vary with the individual. If you have difficulty in locating them in your particular case, you should consult an acupuncturist and get him to tell you where they are. Normally, ear and body acupressure should be alternated daily, the frequency and duration depending on the intensity of the phantom pains. In general, five to ten minutes massage in the evening is adequate.

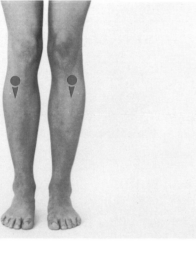

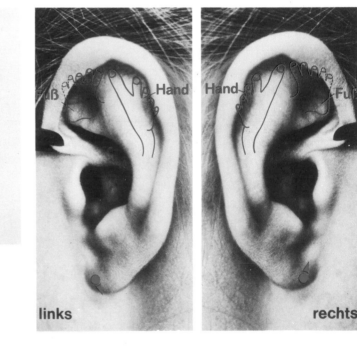

links   rechts

123

Prostate-gland, inflammation of the

The male prostate gland, which is about the size and shape of a chestnut, is situated beneath the bladder. The urethra passes through the middle of it. Inflammation of the prostate is a very unpleasant complaint, which is not always cleared up by the usual forms of treatment, and acupressure is especially helpful in cases such as these.

What are the symptoms?

Some men get a dull pain and sometimes a feeling of discomfort in the general area, rather than pain in the prostate itself, while others may also have a feeling of inflammation in the urethra and a greater need to pass water.

What are the causes?

The most usual cause of irritation or inflammation of the prostate is bacterial infection, but there is often a tendency for the problem to become psychological and so to worsen because of this.

Body acupressure

The main point is the *san-yin-chiao*, three to four finger-widths above the inner ankle-bone, on the edge of the shin, which should be massaged firmly in an upward direction. Next, the *t'ai-ch'ung* point, three finger-widths above the crease between the big toe and second toe, a little towards the big toe, should also be massaged upwards.

The more local 'energy-point' is the *ch'i-hai*, two to three finger-widths (four to five if you are fat) below the navel; massage it upwards. The point for psychological relief is the *tsu-san-li*, on the lower leg, directly beneath the tip of your ring finger when the palm of the hand is rested on the kneecap. Massage this point strongly in a downward direction.

Ear acupressure

On the right ear, the 'point of the prostate' lies in the fold behind the rising front edge, and this should be massaged firmly in an upward

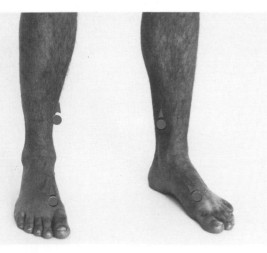

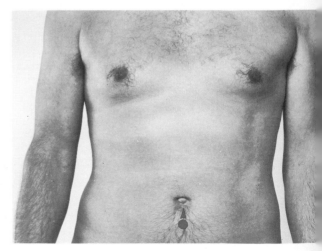

direction. The main psychological point for all thought activity is in the lower front part of the lobe, while the psychological point of relief is situated higher up, just in front of the place where the ear grows out from the head. Massage both these points firmly upwards. On the left ear, use the same points, but reverse the directions of massage.

Treatment

Ear and body acupressure should be alternated daily; five to ten minutes a day is usually enough. Do not reduce your dosage of drugs or medicines except in consultation with your doctor.

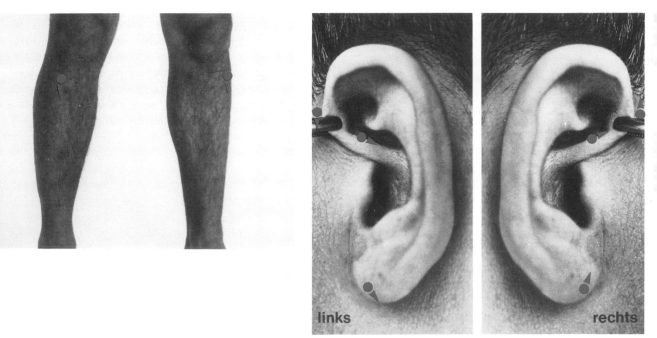

links   rechts

Sciatica

The sciatic nerve is the thickest single nerve cord in the body, about as thick as your little finger. It is at its most vulnerable where it emerges from the spinal column.

What the the symptoms?

The complaint usually begins with frequent attacks of lumbago – muscle stress in the region of the lumbar vertebrae – followed by a slight inflammation of the root of the sciatic nerve, and finally sciatica itself. In this case, the patient gets sharp pains which shoot from the lumbar vertebrae down to the calf or even the ankle.

What are the causes?

Sciatica is usually due to a worn disc in the heavily loaded part of the lower spinal column. The nerve cord emerges from the spine between two vertebrae, through an opening which must not become constricted, but cold and damp can cause cramp in the back muscles which, combined with other harmful effects, compresses the vertebrae and leaves less room for the nerve to pass through. Treatment is by injections, and if these are combined with acupressure, in consultation with your doctor, the inflammation and the cramp will rapidly disappear.

Body acupressure

The principal body points are the *shang-chiao,* in the first hollow of the sacrum (the central bone of the pelvis), which you can feel, and the *tsen-chiao,* in the second hollow about two finger-widths lower down. Massage both points downwards. Next, the *chi'eng-fu* point, at the centre of the crease between the buttock and the thighs, should be massaged downwards.

If the pain goes down to the lower leg and beyond, you should also massage the *wei-chung* point, in the middle of the fold of the knee; the *fei-yang* point, halfway along a line from the outside of the anklebone to the crease at the side of the knee; and the *k'un-lun* point, in the hollow between the outer anklebone and the achilles tendon. Massage all three in a downward direction.

The last two points are *huan-tiao,* which is slightly behind the projecting point of the upper

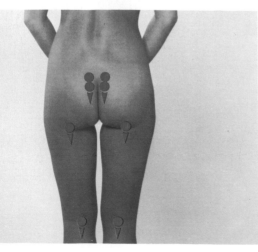

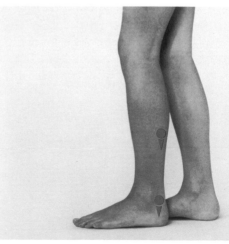

end of the thighbone when you are standing up, and *yang-ling-ch'üan,* just below and in front of the upper end of the fibula (outer legbone). Massage both points downwards.

Ear acupressure

Inflammation of the sciatic nerve is usually felt only on one side, so although ear and body acupressure should be applied on both sides of the body, the points on the painful side should be massaged more firmly. The point for sciatica on the ear is on the forward, upper flat part of the ear, just short of the point where it is obscured by the rising central ridge. This should be massaged forwards, towards the fold.

The central 'energy point', which lies on the ridge where it emerges from the central hollow, should be massaged upwards, and there is another point on the rim of the ear, level with the 'sciatica point', which should also be massaged upwards. The directions of massage given above apply to the right ear; reverse them for the left ear.

Treatment

Ear and body acupressure should be alternated daily. Rest the spine during the period of treatment (no carrying, stooping or gardening), and above all keep it warm. With improvement, you may gradually reduce your intake of prescribed drugs, but only in consultation with your doctor.

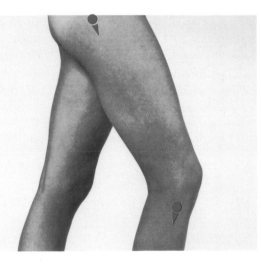

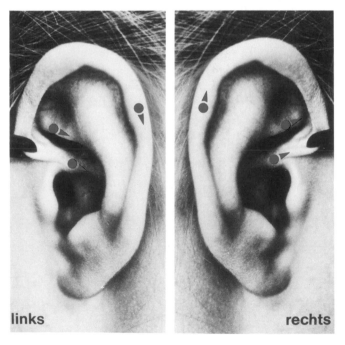

links　　　　　　　　　　　　rechts

127

Sex – stimulating sexual activity

Sexual problems seem to be increasing all the time, from impotence in men to frigidity in women. Acupressure is beneficial in both cases.

What are the symptoms?

Impotence in man either prevents him getting an erection or causes him to ejaculate prematurely. Frigidity in a woman means that she fails to have an orgasm.

What are the causes?

In the great majority of cases, the basic cause of sexual problems is psychological. It is possible for an organic illness to be responsible, such as a disease of the spinal cord, a hormonal disturbance or a drug addiction of some sort (to morphine for example).

If you suspect that your problem is organically based, you should visit an appropriate specialist. However, as most of these problems are of a psychological nature, help is usually obtained from a psychologist, psychotherapist, or marriage-guidance counsellor. As soon as the problem has been identified, acupressure can be started in conjunction with any other form of treatment recommended.

Body acupressure

In the main, the treatment is one of stimulation and energy giving. The key point is the *ch'i-hai*, which has two meanings, 'sea of energy' and 'sea of potency'. It is situated two to three (on fat people, three to four) finger-widths below the navel, and should be massaged in combination with the *kuan-yüan* point, about one hand-width (on fat people, one and a half) above the prominent pubicbone. Massage both points upwards, as strongly as possible.

The *shang-chiao* point is near the base of the spine and lies in a noticeable hollow in the sacrum (central bone of the pelvis). This should be massaged downwards. The *ming-men* ('gateway to life') point, between the second and third dorsal vertebrae, should be massaged upwards.

The 'psychology point', which stimulates the

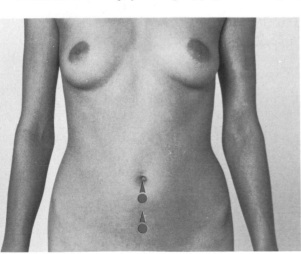

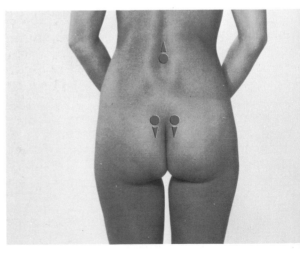

heart and psyche, is situated near the lower corner of the little fingernail, on the side nearest the ring finger. Massage this just below the nail, towards the outside of the hand. Combine this point with the *tsu-san-li,* on the lower leg, which should be massaged downwards. It lies directly beneath the tip of the ring finger when the palm of the hand is placed on the kneecap.

Ear acupressure

On the right ear, stimulate the 'hormone points' inside the fold of the rising central ridge, by massaging them upwards. Sexual functions are helped by massaging the outer edge of the ear upwards. Two points with beneficial psycho-

logical effects are the principal 'relaxation point', just in front of the centre of the ear, where it joins the head, and the principal 'thought point' at the lower front edge of the lobe. Massage both points upwards. On the left ear, the directions of massage should be reversed. Pay particular attention to the key nerve point, which is marked with two spots in the illustration.

Treatment

Ear and body acupressure should be alternated daily. As a rule, one treatment lasting five to ten minutes is enough.

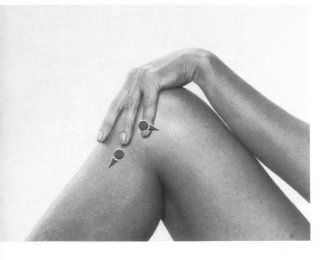

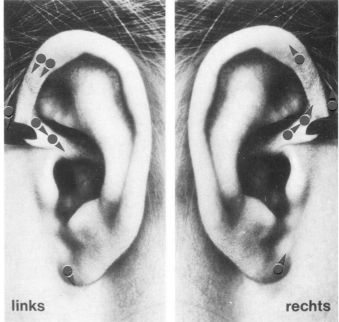

links   rechts

129

Skin allergies and nettle rash

This sort of condition is not usually noticed until the allergy comes out as a reaction to some particular substance or other. In most cases it is neither necessary, nor even advisable, to apply cortisone ointment to the skin. If the doctor prescribes certain drugs, and you apply acupressure as well, the allergy will go more quickly.

What are the symptoms?

Large areas of skin become red, rather like the effects of scarlet fever or measles. Nettle rash usually produces large pimples and all the affected areas itch uncomfortably.

What are the causes?

Allergies are caused by allergens, substances which cause allergic reactions. The difficulty in treating allergies lies in the fact that they vary enormously from individual to individual. With one person it is dog hair, with another strawberries, and with a third certain detergents. In fact, almost anything can produce an allergy, regardless of how the sufferer comes into contact with it, whether from breathing, eating, or simply skin contact (see page 76 for treatment of hay fever). All that can be said is that certain people have strong allergic reactions. Many doctors put this down to a disturbance of the thymus gland, situated behind the upper breastbone. This usually corrects itself in young people, but can be a cause of the complaint in later years.

Body acupressure

The first point to massage is the *ho-ku*, two finger-widths below the knuckle of the index finger and half a finger-width towards the thumb. Massage it towards the elbow. The next is the *ch'üh-ch'ih* which, when the arm is fully bent, lies on the outside of the crease of the elbow. Massage it towards the shoulder. Finally there are two 'change-of-substance' points: the first, called the *wei-chung*, lies in the centre of the fold of the knee. This should be massaged

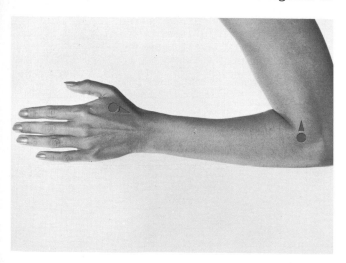

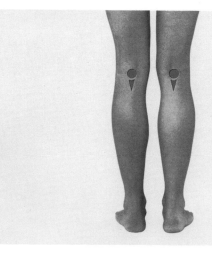

downwards. The second, called the *jan-ku*, is in a little hollow on the inside of the foot, two finger-widths below and the same distance in front of the inner anklebone. This should be massaged towards the anklebone itself.

Ear acupressure

The 'allergy point' lies at the top-centre of the ear. On the right ear, massage this point towards the back of the head, and on the left ear towards the front. You should also massage the 'thymus point', in the middle of the ridge surrounding the central hollow, just above the level at which the forward ridge emerges from the central hollow. The thymus point is massaged downwards on the right ear, upwards on the left.

Treatment

Carry out ear and body acupressure on alternate days, one to three times a day, for five to ten minutes, depending on the severity of the complaint. Try to discover which allergen causes the reaction, and make notes if there appear to be several causes, to try to isolate the real one. It is usually worthwhile to have an allergy test with a skin specialist as well.

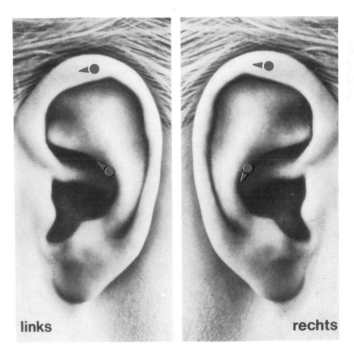

links   rechts

131

Skin irritation

This is only a symptom of a complaint, but is very unpleasant nevertheless. Itching is associated with a sense of pain which is produced by the irritation of the highly sensitive nerve endings of the skin.

What are the symptoms?

An itch is a prickly or smarting sensation on the outer skin layer. In the daytime you can often overcome it by concentrating on something else, but if it comes on in bed at night, an itch can become quite unbearable.

What are the causes?

It needs a doctor to diagnose the cause of a really severe case of itching. It may be due to such things as nervousness, irritating detergents or skin creams, or certain drugs, but there may be a different cause, such as a liver disease or the presence of parasites.

Itching is also associated with all kinds of skin complaints such as nettle rash (see page 130), sores, scars (whether old or recent), and scabs, and with changes in the condition of one's skin, particularly those accompanying children's diseases such as chickenpox, German measles, measles, and scarlet fever. It may be harmless but it can also be dangerous. Acupressure should only be used to relieve the symptom – that is, the itch; the root cause must be diagnosed under proper medical examination.

Body acupressure

The first point is the *ho-ku*, two finger-widths below the knuckle of the index finger and half a finger-width towards the thumb. Massage it in the direction of the elbow. Here you will find the second point, *ch'üh-ch'ih*, which is on the outside of the arm at the base of the crease at the elbow when the arm is fully bent. Massage it upwards.

Next there are two points, the *san-yin-chiao*, three to four finger-widths above the inner point of the ankle, on the edge of the shinbone, and the *tchong-tou*, one hand-width higher and one finger-width to the front. Both should be massaged upwards.

Finally, the *fei-shu* point, which is two finger-widths on each side of the third dorsal vertebra, should be massaged downwards. You can find this by putting your outstretched hand over

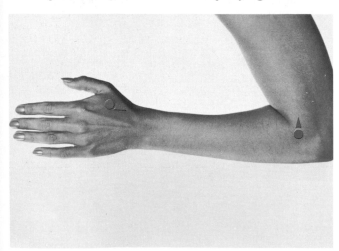

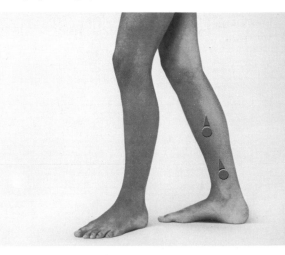

your shoulder near the nape of your neck: the point then lies directly beneath the tip of your middle finger.

Ear acupressure

On the right ear, massage the inner edge of the main circular ridge from top to bottom. The point which releases psychological tension, lying at the upper forward edge of the ear should be massaged upwards, likewise another point at the upper front of the lobe. Reverse these directions on the left ear.

Treatment

Ear and body acupressure should be applied on alternate days, as often as the intensity of the itch demands. This should be done for five to ten minutes at a time. Remember that this only relieves the symptoms of the itch: the root cause must be diagnosed and treated by your doctor. Acupressure, in this case, is a supplementary form of treatment.

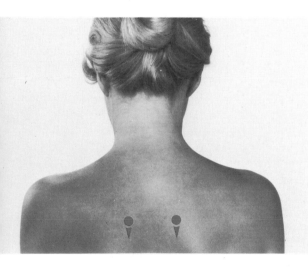

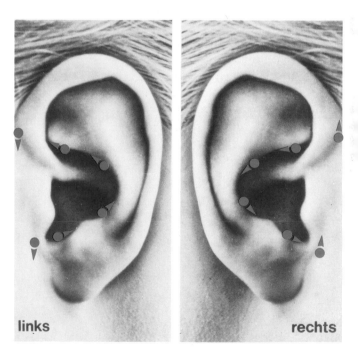

links   rechts

133

Sleeping problems

1 Difficulty in falling asleep

In the Western world we spend millions of pounds every year on sleeping pills, resorting in our thousands to unhealthy 'chemicals' when we are unable to get to sleep naturally. There are two kinds of sleeping problems: getting to sleep, and disturbed sleep. I will deal first with difficulty in falling asleep.

What are the symptoms?

You find that you toss and turn in bed, sometimes for hours on end. You try counting sheep or some other remedy, but nothing helps.

What are the causes?

These are simple enough: your brain's sleep-centre is disturbed by activity in some other part of the brain, which allows you no rest. See your doctor to make sure that it is not due to some other cause, like eating too many rich foods, especially those causing flatulence, before going to bed. He will also be able to say whether the problem is caused by depression, or some other form of psychological or psychosomatic disturbance.

Body acupressure

The principal point used by the Chinese lies exactly midway between the eyebrows, and should be massaged downwards. This is a 'point of rest' according to a tradition which is thousands of years old: it helps you to close your eyes.

Another important point is the *an-mien II*, which lies in a little hollow in the bone behind the ear, just above the hairline. Massage it upwards, applying especially firm pressure on the left side.

One unusual feature of this complaint is that the points on the feet are different for men and women. On a woman, the *chao-hai* point which is one finger-width below the inner anklebone, in a little hollow, should be massaged upwards and backwards. On a man, it is more effective if you massage a point one and a half finger-widths below the outer anklebone, called the

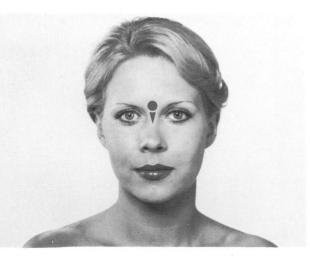

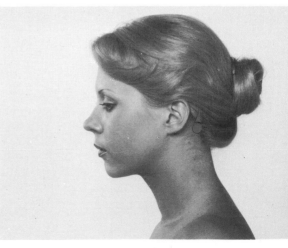

shen-mo. It too lies in a little hollow, near where the skin changes colour from pink to white, and should be massaged towards the toes.

Ear acupressure

The key point, which you can even massage in bed, is easy to find at the back of the lobe. On the right ear, massage this point in an upward and backward direction. The whole area at the front of the ear should be massaged upwards. Reverse the directions on the left ear.

Treatment

Ear and body acupressure should be alternated daily. At first, massage for five to ten minutes each evening before going to bed. Later on, once a week will be enough to prevent a relapse. You can reduce your sleeping pills gradually, by half a tablet at a time, eventually giving them up altogether.

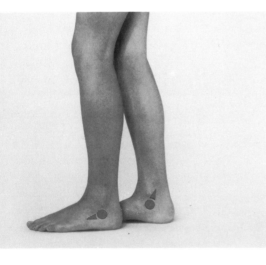

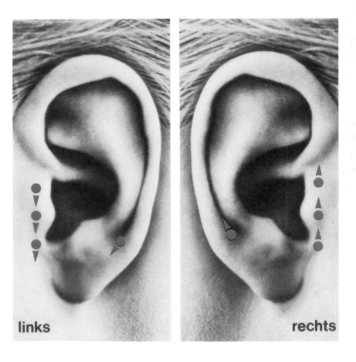

links   rechts

Sleeping problems

2 Disturbed sleep

There are many people who get to sleep relatively easily, only to wake up in the small hours and find themselves unable to drop off again. If you have this problem, try acupressure before going to bed, and again after waking up too soon.

What are the symptoms?

Normally you should sleep right through until morning. As you get older, you need less sleep, but even the elderly generally sleep until five or six o'clock and wake up feeling refreshed. If you suffer from disturbed sleep, however, the situation is totally different. You wake up at three or four in the morning, still feeling tired, and take a sleeping pill to put you to sleep again. Alternatively, you take a strong sedative before you go to bed to guarantee you a full night's sleep.

What are the causes?

As a rule, people with this sort of disturbance also have a complaint of the liver or gall bladder. The Chinese have known for thousands of years that there is a connection between these and the hours of two to four in the morning, and we in the Western world are also aware that gall bladder colic tends to be at its worst at about this time of the night.

Body acupressure

The key point for tension in the liver and gall bladder is the *dang-nang-dian*, three finger-widths below the top of the outer leg bone. There is another point nearby, called the *tsu-san-li*, which lies immediately beneath the tip of the ring finger when you place the palm of your hand on your kneecap. Massage both points downwards, as firmly as possible.

Another important point on the lower leg, called the *tchong-tu*, lies one finger-width backwards and downwards from a point midway between the centre of the kneecap and the inner anklebone. Massage it strongly in an upward direction. Finally, the *tan-chung* point, on the breastbone, level with the male nipples (two

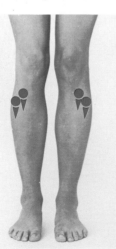
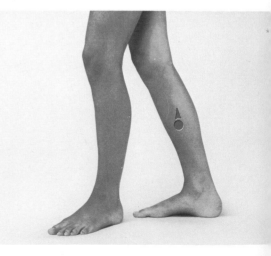

finger-widths below the centre), should be massaged upwards.

Ear acupressure

On the right ear, there is a special 'sleep point' behind the lobe, which should be massaged downwards. It is the exact equivalent of the point on the outside of the lobe, described earlier. Two points which stimulate the activity of the liver and gall bladder, in the central hollow, should be massaged upwards as shown. In general, you need only massage the right ear.

Treatment

Ear and body acupressure should be alternated daily, for five to ten minutes at a time, just before going to bed. Normally, with liver or gall bladder complaints, your doctor will prescribe some form of plant-based medicine, and you should continue with this, as well as your special diet, until you are completely cured.

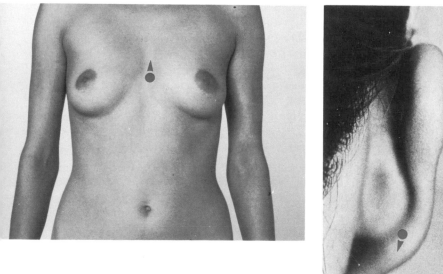

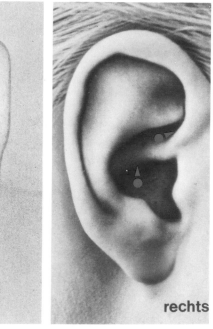

rechts

137

Spinal complaints

1   Disorders of the cervical vertebrae

These are common among people with a sedentary occupation: they usually try to remedy them with massage and various medicaments. In some cases the problem is simply muscular tension, but in others it is more serious, being due to a change in the structure of the spine or vertebral discs. An X-ray is necessary to determine the exact cause.

What are the symptoms?

At first you have a feeling of tension in the neck, which is later followed by pain and restriction in the spine itself, due to tension in the muscles. This is made worse by sitting badly at your desk, or by a depressed state of mind.

What are the causes?

Because the whole spinal column is subject to problems, many doctors believe that it is not really strong enough to support the upright stance and movement of man for any length of time without problems of some sort or other. In other words, as *homo sapiens* developed, his body did not adapt itself properly to walking upright and the consequent loading on the spinal column. His relatively heavy head, which has great freedom of movement, puts a very heavy burden on the cervical vertebrae and the discs between them.

Body acupressure

Begin by massaging the localized points of pain, rubbing outwards, in a star pattern. Next, massage the Chinese points as directed below.

The first point is the *t'ien-shu*, two finger-widths to the side of the centre line of the neck, just above the hairline; the second is the *ta-chu*, two finger-widths to the side of the prominent first thoracic vertebra; and there is another point in this group (not illustrated), which lies exactly halfway between the previous two, and which is very sensitive to pressure.

Next, massage the points *fung-ch'ih*, three finger-widths back from the base of the ear, behind the projecting bone, and just beyond the

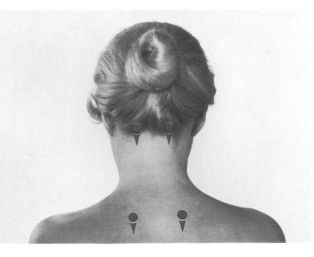

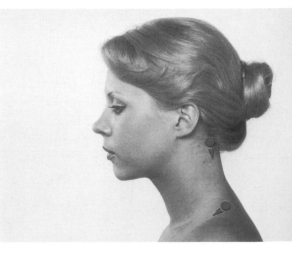

hairline; and the *chien-ching*, one hand-width below the previous point, on the highest part of the shoulder, where the shoulder meets the neck. These points should all be massaged downwards.

The *ta-chui* point, which is just below the prominent seventh cervical vertebra, should be massaged upwards. This also applies to the *ya-men* point, in the middle of the neck, just above the hairline (if you tilt your head backwards you will find a noticeable hollow at this point).

For neck and shoulder pains which are brought on by bad weather, it is especially beneficial to massage the *t'ien-chiao* point, which lies in the middle of an imaginary line between the seventh cervical vertebra and the point of the shoulder; massage it upwards.

Ear acupressure

On the right ear, massage the points for the cervical vertbrae towards the back of the ear, and the pain points of the neck muscles nearby in an upward direction. Also massage the central energy point, on the ridge where it emerges from the central hollow, again in an upward direction. On the left ear the direction of massage should be reversed.

Treatment

Ear and body acupressure should be alternated daily. If you come home from work with a stiff neck, massage the points on the affected side vigorously for five to ten minutes.

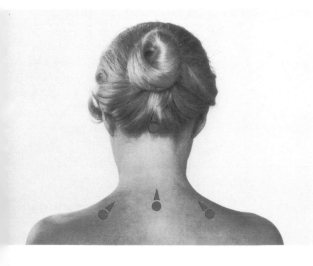

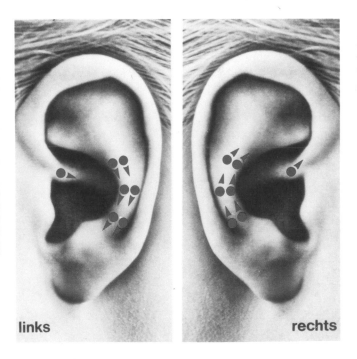

links   rechts

139

Spinal complaints

2 Disorders of the thoracic vertebrae

The twelve thoracic vertebrae, starting immediately below the prominent seventh cervical vertebra, are particularly prone to disorders whether you follow a sedentary occupation or not. Massaging the acupressure points helps to relieve pain in such cases.

What are the symptoms?

A frequent sign of trouble in this area is difficulty in breathing, due to tension and hardening of the muscles, impairing the flexibility of the adjoining ribs. Pains spreading out from the thoracic vertebrae may affect the heart and circulation, or cause cramps in the organs of the chest.

What are the causes?

As mentioned in the previous section, the probable cause is the historical development of man and the fact that he adopted the upright position at an early stage. This spinal column was not strong enough to adapt to the extra burden.

Body acupressure

To start with, massage the localized points of pain, rubbing outwards in a star pattern. You will see what is meant from the examples in the illustration. The key Chinese point for all muscular pains is the *yang-ling-ch'üan*, in a hollow just below and in front of the head of the outer legbone; massage it downwards. This also applies to the *k'un-lun* point, which is particularly effective for the back muscles. This point lies in a hollow between the achilles tendon and the outer anklebone.

Ear acupressure

On the right ear, massage the area for the thoracic vertebrae, above the central hollow, and the area for pains in the back muscles nearby, all in an upward and forward direction. Use a continuous, firm movement. The central energy point, on the ridge where it emerges from the central hollow, should also be massaged upwards. On the left ear, massage the same points, but in the opposite direction.

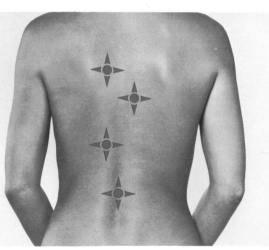

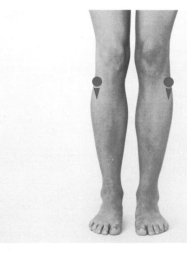

Massage more firmly on the side which hurts most.

Treatment

Ear and body acupressure should be alternated daily. If you come home tense from work and feel pain in the area of the thoracic vertebrae, apply acupressure for five to ten minutes straightaway. Exercise and a hard bed are usually very beneficial.

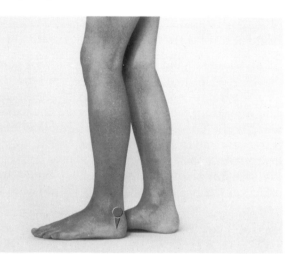

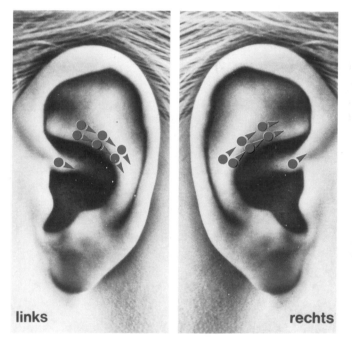

links   rechts

Spinal complaints

3   Disorders of the lumbar vertebrae

Statistics relating to slipped discs, the most common spinal complaint of all, show that the lumbar vertebrae, and particularly the disc between the fourth and fifth bones, are the worst affected of all the three sections of the spinal column.

What are the symptoms?

Initially you think you are getting occasional attacks of lumbago, but you tend to ignore them because they go away of their own accord. However, as you get older, and the wearing process of the spine develops, the localized pains get noticeably sharper. If there is something wrong with the nerve roots, you feel sharp pains in the lower back, and there is widespread pain in this area if the sciatic nerve becomes inflamed (see page 126).

What are the causes?

While the sacrum and the pelvis are firmly joined together to withstand loads, the lumbar vertebrae, which have considerable freedom of movement forwards, have to bear the main burden of the body, and it is their mobility which gives rise to all the problems connected with them.

Body acupressure

Begin by massaging the localized points of pain on the body, rubbing outwards in a star pattern. The illustration shows some typical examples. The important Chinese point for all muscular pains is the *yan-ling-ch'üan,* in the hollow just below and in front of the head of the outer legbone; massage it downwards. This applies to the *k'un-lun* point, which has a very beneficial effect on the back muscles. This point lies in a hollow between the achilles tendon and the outer anklebone.

Ear acupressure

On the right ear, massage the area for the lumbar vertebrae, above the central hollow at

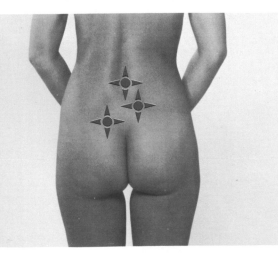

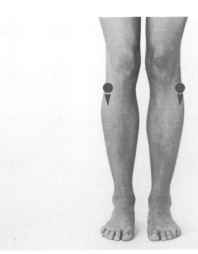

the front of the ear, and the area for pains in the back muscles nearby. Massage them in a forward direction as strongly as possible. The central energy point, on the ridge where it emerges from the central hollow, should be massaged firmly upwards. On the left ear, massage the same points, but in the opposite direction. Massage more firmly on the side which hurts most.

Treatment

Ear and body acupressure should be alternated daily. If you come home tense from work and feel pain in the area of the lumbar vertebrae, apply acupressure for five to ten minutes straightaway. Exercise and a hard bed are usually very beneficial.

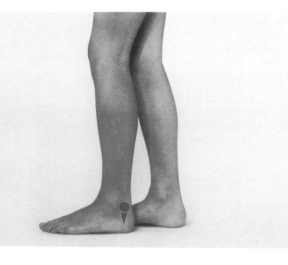

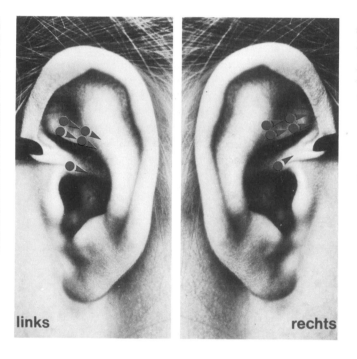

links   rechts

Spinal complaints

4 Pains in the area of the sacrum and coccyx (the base of the spine)

The sacrum consists of five vertebrae joined together to form one large, strong bone. As such, it is not prone to trouble. It forms a substantial part of the pelvic girdle and transfers the weight of the trunk to the pelvis and thereby downwards to the legs. At the top, the sacrum is broad and thick; at the bottom, narrow and thin. Its uppermost surface is connected as a joint to the fifth lumbar vertebra, and this point is the most common of all for spinal problems.

The coccyx is attached to the lower end of the sacrum. It consists of four or five small, individual vertebrae which, by adulthood, have fused together to form one bone. The sacrum and the coccyx can be compressed at the point of contact when sitting down, or if the area is bruised.

What are the symptoms?

Disorders such as a worn disc between the lumbar vertebrae and the sacrum may simply result in localized pain in the area, but if the nerve roots are badly affected the consequences may well be an inflamed sciatic nerve (see 'Sciatica', page 126).

This section will only deal with disorders in the area between the sacrum and the coccyx. Bruising and compressing of the coccyx cause pain which is most noticeable when you sit down and put a load on the injured area. This pain can be remarkably persistent.

What are the causes?

The coccyx is curved like a cuckoo's beak, hence its official medical name *os coccygis*. Because of its shape, the injury caused by any blow is always transmitted to the point where it connects with the sacrum, its weakest point.

Body acupressure

First, massage the localized points of pain, rubbing outwards in a star pattern. The Chinese point associated directly with the junction of the sacrum and coccyx is the *yao-shu*. This lies immediately on the junction itself, and should

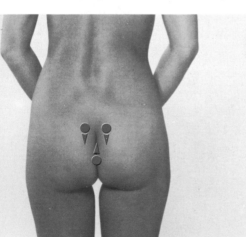

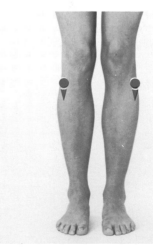

be massaged upwards. The point of general importance for the sacrum is the *chang-chiao,* in the first noticeable hollow in the sacrum itself; massage it downwards.

For muscular tension massage the *yang-ling-ch'uan* point, in the hollow just below and in front of the head of the outer legbone, in a downward direction. This also applies to the *k'un-lun* point, in a hollow between the achilles tendon and the outer anklebone.

Ear acupressure

On the right ear, the area in the upper front corner, which is normally overlapped and obscured by the rising outer rim, should be massaged upwards and forwards. Also massage the general energy point, on the ridge, where it emerges from the central hollow, in an upward direction. On the left ear, massage the same points, but in the opposite directions.

Treatment

Ear and body acupressure should be alternated daily, for five to ten minutes at a time.

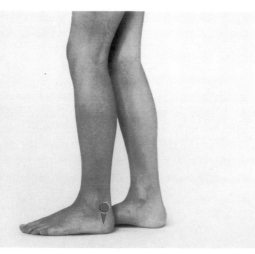

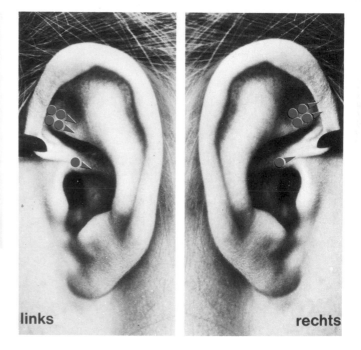

links   rechts

145

Stomach pains and gastric or peptic ulcers

Stomach complaints, which are very common, are due to irritation or inflammation of the lining of the stomach. Acupressure is very suitable for all complaints of this nature.

What are the symptoms?

Stomach pains occur in various forms. In some cases pain is felt more or less continuously, while in others it comes on soon after eating a meal. It generally occurs near the navel, frequently above it and on the right-hand side. A doctor can diagnose inflammation of the stomach lining or a gastric ulcer by X-ray.

What are the causes?

The pains are due to an inflammation in the lining of the stomach or duodenum, properly known as gastritis or duodenitis. In severe cases the lining becomes eroded, resulting in an ulcer. There are several causes for complaints of this nature, such as the irritant effect of certain kinds of food or drink, or the over-production of hydrochloric acid in the stomach through nervous impulses. The latter can be brought on by periods of stress, anger, or jealousy.

Body acupressure

The *t'ai-i* point lies three finger-widths above and a similar distance to the side of the navel, and should be massaged downwards. The *shang-kuan* point, two finger-widths above the halfway point between the navel and the breastbone, should be massaged upwards. The *tan-chung* point, which is halfway up the breastbone, level with the male nipples, should also be massaged upwards. (This point is also used for heartburn.)

Other important points for the stomach are the *tsu-san-li,* which is on the lower leg, directly beneath the ring finger when the palm of the hand is placed on the kneecap, and *chü-hsü-hsia-lien,* which is three finger-widths below the halfway point on a line from the centre of the kneecap to the outer anklebone. This point has a direct effect on the small intestine, and is used

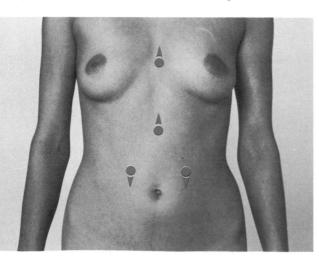

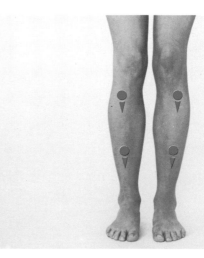

for duodenal pains and ulcers. Massage both these points downwards.

Finally, the points *hsing-chien*, in the crease between the big toe and second toe, slightly towards the big toe, and *t'ai-ch'ung*, three finger-widths higher up, should both be massaged upwards.

Ear acupressure

The most important point, which affects the nerve centre of the whole solar plexus, is on the right ear, at the base of the outer rim where it emerges from the central hollow. Massage it strongly upwards and forwards. For this complaint, the other two points are supplementary. They lie just above and below the first, and should be massaged in a clockwise direction. Massage the same points on the left ear in the opposite direction.

Treatment

In these cases, ear acupressure is particularly effective, so do this two days running, followed by one day of body acupressure. Keep to your diet, and only reduce your dosage of drugs or medicines in consultation with your doctor.

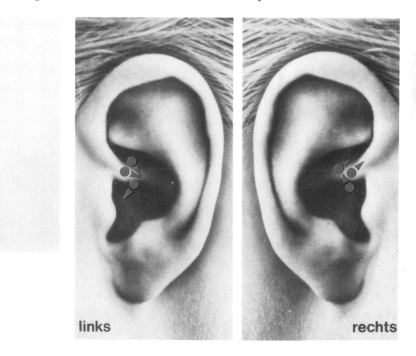

links   rechts

Stuttering

This is a psychological speech disturbance which usually starts when a child goes to school for the first time, or at the onset of puberty, particularly with boys. It sometimes passes as the child develops. Acupressure is very beneficial in cases of stuttering. The child should learn to apply acupressure himself.

What are the symptoms?

For fluent speech you need a combination of correct breathing, articulation, and phonation (the production of vocal sounds), and a defect in any of these functions can cause hesitation over pronouncing certain sounds or syllables.

What are the causes?

While it is possible for a physical deformation to play a part, the problem is essentially psychological, which means that stuttering may be due to almost any form of bad psychological experience, such as fear or anxiety (especially the anxiety of waiting), being in conflict or having a difficult upbringing, or being the victim of impatience, abuse, or teasing. At three or four, a child's mental development may be in advance of his ability to speak.

Body acupressure

The first point, the *ch'eng-chiang*, is in the little hollow between the lower lip and the chin and should be massaged upwards. Next the *chiu-wei* point, at the base of the breastbone, should also be massaged upwards. In combination with these, massage the *hou-ting* point, which lies in a little hollow in the centre of the skull, two and a half to three finger-widths behind an imaginary line joining the ears. Massage it towards the forehead.

The *tung-li* point, two to three finger-widths above the base of the palm in line with the little finger, should be massaged towards the latter, and the psychological relief point, the *tsu-san-li*, should be massaged downwards. You will find this beneath the tip of your ring finger, on your lower leg, when you place the palm of your hand on your kneecap.

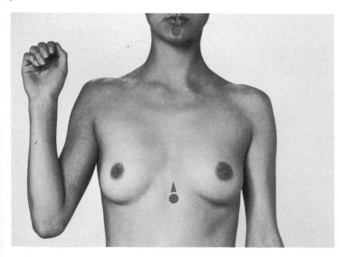

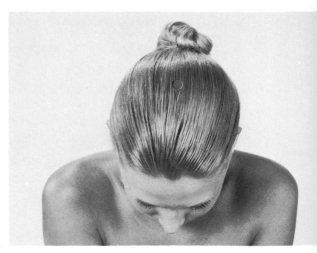

Ear acupressure

On the right ear, the psychological relief point, which is situated in the upper front edge, where the ear joins the head, should be massaged firmly upwards. There is another point associated with the brain, just inside the lowest part of the central hollow, and this should be massaged outwards and towards the top of the lobe. On the left ear, massage in the opposite direction in each case, and with less pressure.

Treatment

The child should be taught to apply acupressure to himself, and should alternate ear and body acupressure daily, once or twice a day, for five to ten minutes at a time. Parents should make sure this has been done.

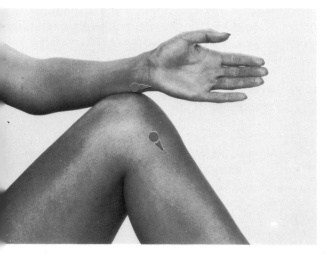

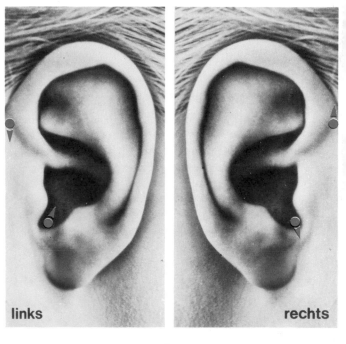

links   rechts

Tennis elbow

Tennis elbow, as it is generally called, is a painful inflammation in the area of the elbow joint, at the base of the upper armbone, which can occur on the inside or outside or even on both sides of the arm. It is common among painters, woodworkers, gardeners, porters, and of course tennis players.

What are the symptoms?

You feel pain in the upper part of the elbow, usually on the outside and especially when you move your hand and fingers, but pain can also be caused by pressure on the affected area.

What are the causes?

It is usually due to irritation or inflammation in places where the tendons have attached themselves to the bone. The reason for this is strain from over-exertion or repeated injury. Sometimes there may also be a defect in the cervical vertebrae (the top of the spinal column), which causes interference and impedes recovery. In this case, acupressure treatment for tennis elbow should be combined with that for the spinal column (see page 138). A medical examination will show if this is necessary.

Body acupressure

The first point, the *ch'üh-ch'ih,* will be found at the outer end of the elbow crease, when the arm is fully bent. It should be massaged upwards. Next, the *san-li* point, on the outside of the forearm, three to four finger-widths below the previous point (on an imaginary line to the forefinger) should also be massaged upwards. The *ch'ih-tse* point, in the middle of the elbow crease, should be massaged in the direction of the hand.

The *wan-ku* point, which lies in a hollow on the outside edge of the wrist, and *wai-kuann* point, on the back of the arm midway between the tip of the middle finger and the point of the elbow, should both be massaged towards the elbow. Finally, the *chien-chen* point should be massaged upwards. To find this, let your arm hang down, then search for a small hollow two finger-widths above the crease at the back of the armpit.

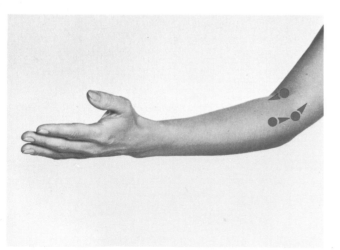

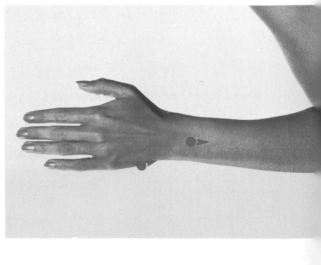

Ear acupressure

On the right ear, the pain point for the elbow is just above the centre line of the ear, between the back edge and the central hollow: massage it upwards. At the same level, on the back of the ear, is the motor point for the muscles and joint, and this should also be massaged upwards. If the left elbow is affected, massage the same points on the left ear, in the same direction as on the right – that is, upwards.

Treatment

Ear and body acupressure should be alternated daily, once or twice a day, for five to ten minutes at a time. To prevent a recurrence, do not exert the arm during the course of treatment, and rest the elbow as much as possible.

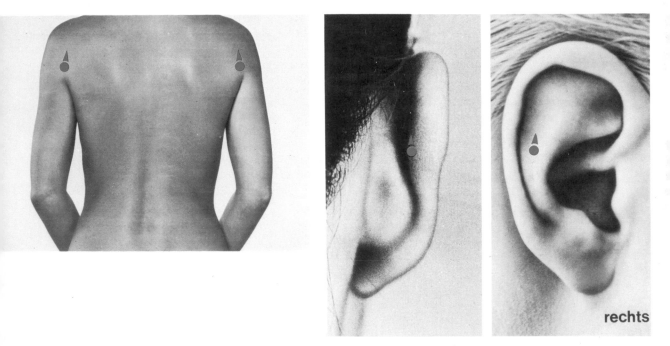

rechts

151

Tonsillitis

In China, acupuncture and acupressure are used in the home to treat simple complaints before they become serious illnesses. Many Europeans are now beginning to see that this makes sense. One complaint to which such treatment particularly applies is tonsillitis which, in the case of repeated attacks, can lead to rheumatic fever. Needless to say, recurring tonsillitis should be prevented and acupressure helps to do this, as well as to reduce any swelling in the throat when it occurs.

What are the symptoms?

The tonsils lie on each side of the throat. Normally the size of olives, they become almost as big as walnuts when inflamed. The area around them also gets red and swollen.

What is the cause?

Inflammation of the throat, and especially of the tonsils, is often noticed when the cold weather sets in. This part of the throat, like the nose, is the first point in the body's warning system against infection, so it is quite normal for it to redden and get swollen from time to time. It becomes an illness when the swelling is excessive, when pus is discharged, when the tissue splits open, and when it happens several times a year.

Doctors are divided as to treatment. Some advise having the tonsils out, others to leave them, because of their role in the body's warning system. It is at least common sense not to let the complaint get to the stage at which the tonsils discharge matter persistently, which is very bad for the body. Under these circumstances an operation is advisable. But the best thing is to prevent serious tonsillitis altogether, by using acupressure and by wearing scarves, roll-neck pullovers and warm socks when the weather turns cold.

Body acupressure

The first point, the *schao-shang,* at the base of the thumbnail, on the outside, should be massaged inwards, just below the nail. Next, the *ho-ku* point, two finger-widths below the forefinger knuckle and half a finger-width towards the thumb, and the *hau-hsi* point, which has an

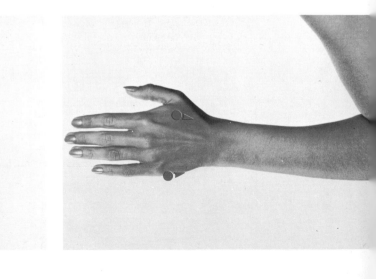

important influence on all mucous membranes, and which lies just below the little finger knuckle on the outside, should both be massaged towards the elbow. Lastly, there is a local point, the *tienn-yong,* which is situated just behind, and one finger-width above, the point of the jaw. Massage it upwards.

Ear acupressure

On the right ear, the 'tonsil point' is towards the back of the lobe; massage it upwards. The central energy point is on the ridge, where it emerges from the central hollow. Massage it upwards and forwards. Reverse the directions on the left ear.

Treatment

Ear and body acupressure should be alternated daily. In acute cases, apply massage one to three times a day, for five to ten minutes at a time. As a preventative measure you need only do this once or twice a week. If the doctor has ordered you to gargle, or has prescribed throat tablets, keep up the treatment until he says otherwise.

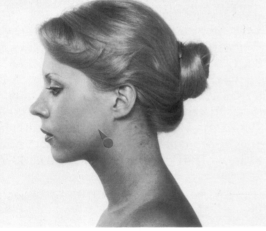

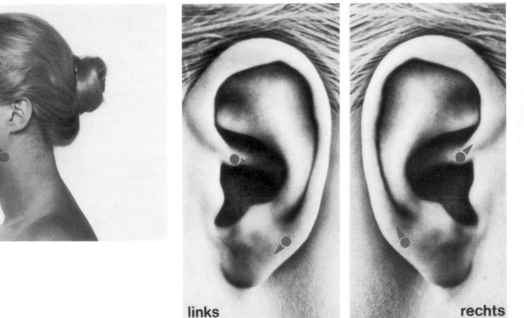

links   rechts

Varicose veins

At first, varicose veins give little discomfort, but later on you may get a heavy feeling in the leg and 'tugging', cramping pains. Sometimes the ankles swell up too. In severe cases it is important to wear supporting bandages or elastic stockings. It may even be advisable to have an operation to have the veins sealed or removed altogether. Acupressure cannot repair varicose veins, but it is beneficial in relieving the accompanying pains in the leg.

What are the symptoms?

Varicose veins are veins which have lost their normal shape and tension, and have become swollen (sometimes to finger thickness) and tortuous. They occur in the lower leg, sometimes on the back of the foot, and occasionally in the thigh.

What are the causes?

They are usually due to a weakness in the connecting tissue in the vein, and may be brought on by an increase in back pressure when the blood flow is restricted, which is why so many women suffer from this complaint after pregnancy. I strongly advise all women to wear elastic stockings during pregnancy, especially since they are now almost indistinguishable from nylons or tights.

People who stand all day also tend to get varicose veins; shop assistants, hairdressers, waitresses, and so on. They too should wear elastic stockings; they should also practise acupressure to prevent varicose veins from forming. Men are less inclined to have a weakness in the connecting tissue, and do not suffer from varicosity to the same extent as women do.

Body acupressure

The *shang-ch'in* point, which is the master point for all tissue weaknesses, is very important here. It lies two finger-widths to the front of, and one finger-width below, the centre of the inner anklebone. There is also the *t'ai-chung* point, two to three finger-widths above the crease between the big and second toes, and slightly towards the former. Massage both points upwards. The *k'un-lun* point, in the hollow

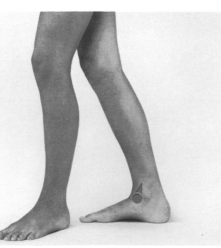
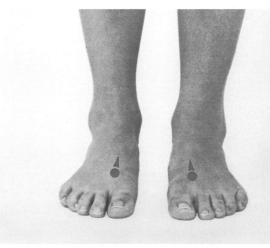

between the achilles tendon and the outer anklebone, should be massaged downwards.

Finally, there is the *tsu-san-li* point, on the lower leg, immediately beneath the ring finger when the palm of the hand is placed on the kneecap so that the middle finger touches the shin. Massage it downwards.

Ear acupressure

There is a row of points lying in the small triangular hollow towards the top, front part of the ear, which should be massaged towards the back on both ears.

Treatment

Acupressure can do no more than relieve or remove the symptoms – the discomfort – of varicose veins. If you wear elastic stockings, continue to do so. Carry out ear and body acupressure on alternate days, as often and for as long as the severity of the complaint demands.

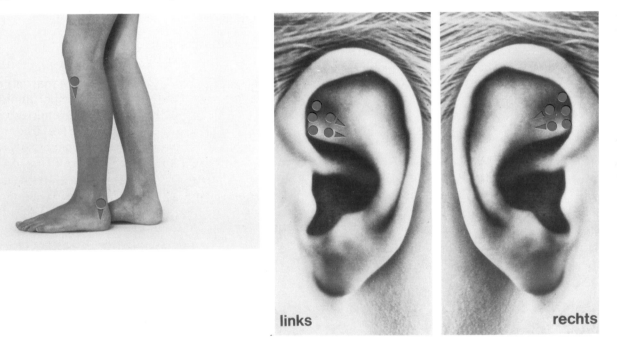

links   rechts

155

Vertigo (Giddiness) – a symptom of many illnesses

Some of the conditions which give rise to giddiness are high or low blood pressure, bad circulation, complaints of the ear and cerebellum (lower part of the brain), and food poisoning. It can also be a sign of an infectious illness, or of several forms of heart disease, of persistent, though negligible, loss of blood, or of a weakness in the adrenal, pituitary, or thyroid glands.

It is impossible to cover all the illnesses which can give rise to giddiness in this book, so I have chosen three which can be treated fairly simply by acupressure. Obviously, only a doctor can diagnose the cause of giddiness in your particular case: he will also be able to advise you whether acupressure is a suitable form of treatment.

1 Circulation problems

When you get up, your circulation has to adjust itself to the body's needs during the day ahead. You may find that yours responds very slowly, or functions inadequately if you stand for any length of time. The result is that your head starts to swim or feel somehow 'empty', or you are overcome by giddiness or nausea.

What are the symptoms?

You seem to lose your sense of balance, as if the floor were swaying beneath your feet.

What are the causes?

Circulation weaknesses may be due to such things as blood disease, hormonal disturbances, heart complaints, or infectious illnesses. As a rule, a combination of medical treatment and acupressure should be effective.

Body acupressure

The principal Chinese point is the *ch'i-hai* ('sea of energy'), two to three (if you are fat, four or

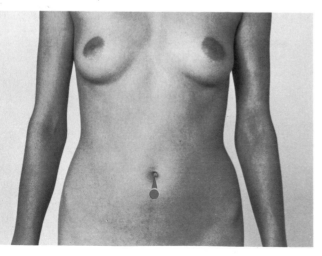

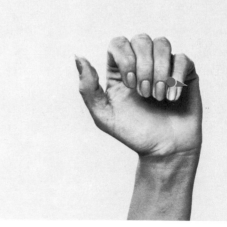

five) finger-widths below the navel. Massage it firmly upwards. Next, the stimulation point for the heart, the *shao-chong*, near the inside lower corner of the little fingernail, should be massaged across the finger, below the nail, from the inside out. Lastly, the stimulation point for the circulation, the *chung-ch'ung*, which is near the lower corner of the middle fingernail, next to the index finger, should be massaged across the finger below the nail and towards the ring finger.

Ear acupressure

On the right ear, the 'central energy point', on the ridge where it emerges from the central hollow, should be massaged firmly upwards. There is another point, low down in the central hollow, which should be massaged in an upward and backward direction. It is not possible to show its position clearly in the illustration, as it is partly obscured by a slight

bulge in the lower ridge. The last point is in front of the top of the lobe, and this should be massaged firmly upwards. On the left ear the points are the same, but the directions of massage should be reversed.

Treatment

Ear and body acupressure should be alternated daily, one to three times a day, for five to ten minutes, depending on the severity of the complaint. You must visit your doctor if you have attacks of giddiness; this is very important. If the cause is high blood pressure, there are other points for acupressure, which an acupuncturist will show you, once he has established the root cause of the problem.

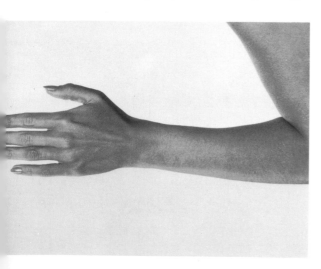

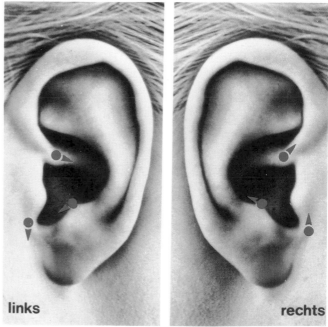

links   rechts

Vertigo (Giddiness)

2 Functional disturbance of the cerebellum

Acupressure is very beneficial in relieving this type of disturbance.

What are the symptoms?

The cerebellum, which is the lower part of the brain, is responsible for co-ordinating all the body's movements. To do this, it acts on the messages it receives from a number of sources – the balance mechanism in the inner ear, the body's motor system, and the sense organs. If the cerebellum fails to do its job properly, you feel giddy and start to sway about, walk unsteadily, and find that instead of pointing directly at a particular object, you point past it.

What are the causes?

'Cerebellum vertigo' may be due to a tumour, a haemorrhage or a circulation failure (or even have its origins in the upper spinal column). A neuro-specialist should carry out an examination and diagnose the true cause. Carry out acupressure in consultation with him.

Body acupressure

The first point is the *t'ien-chu,* two finger-widths to the side of the middle of the neck, just above the hairline. The other point is the *feng-ch'ih,* three finger-widths back from the prominent bone behind the ear and just above the hairline. Both points should be massaged downwards.

Ear acupressure

This is particularly effective. The point for the cerebellum lies in the hollow behind the ear and should be massaged downwards on the right ear, upwards on the left.

Treatment

Ear and body acupressure should be alternated daily, for five to ten minutes at a time. The treatment should be supervised by your neuro-specialist.

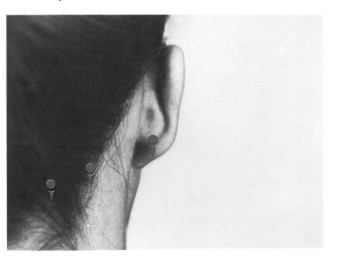

Vertigo (Giddiness)

3   Functional disturbance in the ear

This complaint, properly known as otogenous (of the ear) vertigo, almost always occurs as a 'spinning sensation'. It is due to poor circulation, or inflammation or infection of the semi-circular canals inside the ear, and for this reason you should only carry out acupressure in consultation with your E.N.T. (ear, nose and throat) specialist.

What are the symptoms?

You feel as if your sense of balance has been disturbed: the floor sways, or everything spins; you may even have a tendency to fall down. You may also experience difficulty in hearing, buzzing in the ears, of involuntary movements of the eyeballs (nystagmus).

What are the causes?

As there are so many potential causes, you should get your E.N.T. specialist to give you an examination and diagnosis to establish the cause of your particular complaint, and then practise acupressure in consultation with him.

Ear acupressure

There is one key point, the 'point of the labyrinth of the ear'. This is behind the ear, fairly high up in the valley. Massage it downwards on the right ear, upwards on the left. No other point on the ear or the body is as effective as this particular one.

Treatment

Massage the point described as strongly as possible, on both ears. Now and then, apply the acupressure for stimulating the ear functions (see page 158) on alternate days.

rechts   links

Addresses

You can obtain the names and addresses of medically qualified acupressure practitioners from the following:

British Medical Acupuncture Society
(Dr Julian N Kenyon)
21 Aidburth Drive, Sefton Park,
Liverpool L17 4JQ

American Academy for Acupuncture
& Auricular Medicine
(Michael Graf, M.D.)
1634 Gull Road, Kalamazoo
Michigan 49001, USA

North Amercian Academy for Acupuncture
Research
(Dr L S McKibbin)
Box 28, Wheatly Ontario
NOP 2 PO Canada

Australian Acupuncture Society
(Dr I Schneideman)
Beky Park, Forest Glen,
4555 Queensland
Australia

For other countries, the addresses of qualified practitioners can be obtained from local or national medical associations.